THE BREAKTHROUGH JOURNAL

Flower Edition

BETH BIANCA

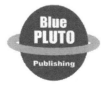

Blue
PLUTO
Publishing

The Breakthrough Journal: Flower Edition / Beth Bianca --1st ed.

ISBN-10: 0-692-94693-4

ISBN-13: 978-0-692-94693-0

Join Beth Bianca's motivational community, using your phone.

Text **LIVING** to **444999.**

Meet Beth Bianca online at: **BethBianca.com**

Also written by Beth Bianca.

Mindset Breakthrough: *Achieve Weight-Loss Surgery Success*

The Breakthrough Journal: *Butterfly Edition*

TABLE OF CONTENTS

INTRODUCTION

Weight-loss surgery is NOT the easy way out. Sadly, there are too many bariatric patients searching for answers to why they can't lose more weight. Or, wondering why they've regained some or all of their weight.

Successful bariatric patients have two things in common. They know what to do, and they have the mindset to do what they know. Unsuccessful bariatric patients don't know the basics; or, even more difficult to overcome, they don't do what they know.

That's why I created The Breakthrough Journal. I've lost 229 pounds during my bariatric journey. Now I'm passionate about helping other bariatric patients. I yo-yo dieted my entire adult life until I ended up weighing 394 pounds. I was riddled with health issues and was housebound, unable to walk without help. I had a Vertical Sleeve Gastrectomy in April of 2015. The hardest part of my journey was not the surgery; instead, it was dealing with all the old, life-long thoughts and behaviors I had about food. I'm sorry to say those old thoughts and behaviors were not removed during surgery.

The Breakthrough Journal is based on what I know works and is backed with research. First, I'll explain, in a concise and easy to understand manner, the Bariatric Basics I used to lose 229 pounds. Then you'll be guided, step-by-step, to choosing your personal Breakthrough Goal. This Breakthrough Goal will lay the foundation for creating the biggest, positive change to your life. And, it doesn't stop there. The Breakthrough Journal will be your accountability companion. For the next 12 weeks it will keep you focused on your plan and help you achieve your Breakthrough Goal. All while making your transformation fun and rewarding at the same time.

If you follow what this journal shows you, step by step, at the end of 12 weeks you will accomplish your life-changing goal and create habits for long-term success. Don't be the person who stays stuck wondering how people achieve weight-loss surgery success. Be the person who reaches your goals and inspires others with your transformation. Be the person who is confident and does what needs to be done. Be the person who knows you can accomplish anything you desire.

THE BREAKTHROUGH JOURNAL

It's all here. This journal is a blueprint for making the permanent changes necessary for permanent results. Take control and enjoy the life you were meant to live. All you need to do is turn the page and get started. If I did it, so can you!

A MAGICAL SECRET?

What if I said a specific action, when done consistently, could double your weight loss and help keep it off?

What if this very same action could burn more calories than exercise?

This all sounds like the weight loss claims we've heard for decades, doesn't it?

What is this magical secret? It's no secret at all. This amazing action is simply keeping a food journal. Yes, we've all heard that before. But, how many people really do track their food? Well, it appears people who've been successful with losing weight have done so.

In a study reported on WebMd.com [Ref-1], Victor Stevens, Ph.D., senior investigator at Kaiser Permanente Center for Health Research, says, "Those who kept food records six days a week -- jotting down everything they ate and drank on those days -- lost about twice as much weight as those who kept food records one day a week or less." That alone should make you want to pick up a pen and start tracking your food.

In an article on Fooducate.com [Ref-2], Yoni Freehoff, MD says, "Food diaries burn more calories than exercise - sort of. It's far easier to not eat calories than it is to burn them. Figure it takes most people nearly an hour of vigorous exercise to burn 500 calories. Those same folks can likely find, trim and remove 500 daily calories from their diets by keeping a food diary - an effort that will take 5 minutes at most."

I can testify to the previous statement. During my six-month pre-op stage, I was so ill I could no longer walk or do any normal activity. Yet, I was able to lose 59 pounds just sitting in a chair and sleeping in my bed. My activity level was a big, fat zero. I lost the weight by tracking my food and staying within my nutrition requirements.

After I realized there wasn't a magic pill for weight loss, I thought exercise was the key to losing weight. A major "ah-ha" moment came from my doctor. She was explaining how losing weight would improve my health conditions. I was perplexed. Looking at her I said, "I can't even walk, how can I exercise?" She looked me straight in the eye and said that I could lose weight without exercising. The look on my face must have been like I saw a ghost. I was in complete shock.

That was the first time in my life that someone said it's possible to lose weight without exercising. And, it came from my doctor. Talk about a major light-bulb moment. That was the beginning of a whole new life for me. I've been tracking my food ever since. Now, I've lost 229 pounds; and I will continue to track my food for the rest of my life. It's really not hard to do, and the benefits are amazing.

So, now you know why tracking food is important. Are you ready to commit to keeping a food journal on a consistent, daily basis?

COLORING PAGES TOO!

Coloring books have become quite popular in recent years. Once thought of as an activity for children, now adults are experiencing amazing benefits from coloring.

In an article at MedicalDaily.com [Ref-3], Dr. Stan Rodski, a neuropsychologist says, "Coloring elicits a relaxing mindset, similar to what you would achieve through meditation. Like meditation, coloring allows us to switch off our brains from other thoughts and focus on the moment."

The article continues with Dr. Joel Pearson, a brain scientist at the University of New South Wales in Australia, pointing out that "Concentrating on coloring an image may facilitate the replacement of negative thoughts and images with pleasant ones." Do you think that might help at the end of a busy, stressful day?

Dr. Pearson continues, "You have to look at the shape and size, you have to look at the edges, and you have to pick a color . . . It should occupy the same parts of the brain that stops any anxiety-related mental imagery happening as well. . . Anything that helps you control your attention is going to help."

Coloring is a great way to deal with food cravings and head hunger too. You can color instead of dealing with impulse food desires. Coloring will change your focus away from food to picking the best-colored pencil to complete your image.

In the Huffington Post [Ref-4], Dr. Nikki Martinez, Psy.D. LCPC, says, "For many, boredom, lack of structure, and stress are the greatest triggers they have. . . The time and focus that adult coloring takes helps the individual remove the focus from the negative issues and habits, and focus them in a safe and productive way."

We've all seen advice about dealing with food cravings. There's someone who says wait five minutes to see if the craving passes. And, another person who says try exercising instead. I know those suggestions never worked for me. Really? The last thing I wanted to do was exercise while having a food craving. And waiting five minutes? That just kept me focused on the food I wanted. Yeah, five minutes passed; and I was absolutely, positively sure that I wanted to have the food.

What worked for me was replacing the food cravings with something more enjoyable and easy to do. That's when I first heard about adult coloring and its benefits. I wish I had known about it sooner, but better late than never.

These are the reasons I decided to add coloring pages to each day of The Breakthrough Journal. While working on your Breakthrough Goal and creating new habits, coloring will become part of your new routine. It will clear your mind of stress, keep your focus away from bad behaviors, and give you something fun to do along the way.

THE BARIATRIC BASICS

There are two ingredients to a successful weight-loss surgery journey. First, you need to know the "Bariatric Basics." Second, you need to use them consistently for the rest of your life

As we begin with the Bariatric Basics, I want to stress the importance of following the specific instructions given to you by your surgeon. What I am sharing with you are the Bariatric Basics that have worked for me. They were the instructions provided to me during my nutrition classes, which were taught by my bariatric surgery team at a Center of Excellence facility. This has been my blueprint for consistent weight-loss success. If you have gone through nutrition classes, this is intended to be a refresher for you. It is not meant to replace the instructions provided by your surgery team.

1. *Keep a Food Journal* — You must know exactly what you are eating and how often. Every item you eat needs to be logged, including snacks. Total calories for the day should be no more or less than your doctor recommends for your post-op stage. Sometimes keeping a food journal is the first thing people stop doing. I plan on using a food journal for the rest of my life. When you log your food, there is no way for weight-gain to sneak up on you.

2. *Breakfast — Eat something the first 30 minutes after waking up.* In the article titled, "The Half-Hour Window," at RiversideOnline.com" [Ref-5], they explain that when we are sleeping at night our body shifts into a fat storing mode to conserve energy while we sleep. They go on to state, "Eating a meal within 30 minutes of waking will help increase the rate of our metabolism which has slowed down to conserve the stored energy." The article continues, "The longer you wait to eat, the greater the risk your metabolism will slow down and shift into the fat-storing starvation mode." This seems like a pretty simple step to start the day off strong. There is no reason for my metabolism to be sleeping when I have already started my day. Sometimes I have a low-fat cheese stick within 15 minutes of waking up. Then I have my full breakfast an hour later when I have more time.

3. *Protein — Needs vary depending on your post-op stage.* The UCLA's Bariatric Program Material [Ref-6] recommends between 60-90 grams of protein per day. Make sure you do what it takes to meet your protein requirements every day.

4. *Water — Drink 64 oz per day.* This includes the water you mix with protein powder and/or use in decaffeinated tea. After weight-loss surgery, because the size of our stomach has been reduced, it is more difficult for us to get our necessary water intake. We need to be especially careful not to become dehydrated. When consuming beverages, we should avoid caffeine and carbonated drinks. In the Johns Hopkins [Ref-7] bariatric information guide, they explain why: "Carbonation may cause abdominal discomfort and may stretch out your new stomach over time. Caffeine may irritate the stomach and increase your risk for an ulcer after surgery." Another important item to mention is that you should drink all beverages between meals, not during the meal. An article from the Bariatric Surgery Source [Ref-8] states, "You can't drink with your meals and need to wait at least an hour after you eat before drinking anything. If you don't, the liquids will quickly flush the food through your stomach. This can affect digestion, make you feel hungry and lead to weight gain after bariatric surgery."

5. *Vitamins — Always take your doctor's recommended dosage of vitamins.* This is another way to avoid malnutrition and is extremely important for bariatric patients.

6. *Exercise — Get plenty of exercise.* The American Heart Association [Ref-9] recommends, "At least 30 minutes of moderate-intensity aerobic activity at least 5 days per week for a total of 150" minutes per week. I have to admit, since I wasn't even able to walk at the time of my surgery, this is a goal that took some time to reach. Find what exercise works best for you and gradually build your endurance. Any type of exercise is better than none.

7. *Avoid temptation — Don't even try one of your impulse foods or beverages.* Once you open that door, it is hard to close it again. It's definitely not worth the damage that may result from a little indulgence.

I use the following information as my guideline when preparing meals. It helps me to make a good per serving food choice. The meal outline was provided to me by my nutritionist and it has worked well.

• Protein - 10 grams or higher (the higher it is the better)

• Fat - 5 grams or less

• Sugar - 5 grams or less (only exception is skim milk)

WEIGHT-LOSS STALLS

The Scale Isn't Always Your Friend. After my Vertical Sleeve Gastrectomy surgery, I hit a plateau during week six. At this point I had already lost a total of 87 pounds, with only 30 of that being post-surgery. I didn't even think it was possible to have a stall so soon after surgery. I emailed my nutritionist to see if this was normal. She said that it definitely was normal and that, once my body was over it, I would see a jump in lost pounds. She raised my protein up to 88 grams per day. The next week I lost 3.5 pounds.

First and foremost, DO NOT let a scale plateau ever take you off track. Everyone who has ever lost weight has hit a stall at some point. If you have a lot of weight to lose, you will most likely hit more than one stall.

An article at ObesityCoverage.com [Ref-10] describes a plateau as this:

> Your body is constantly seeking something called homeostasis. Homeostasis is a process that maintains the human body's internal environment in response to changes in external conditions. So when food decreases significantly (external condition), your body adjusts internally to create stability (stable weight). So, to counteract the lack of food in your environment, the body slows down your basal metabolic rate – your metabolism slows down and you hit a wall. You haven't changed your eating or exercise habits and you hit a wall before you reach your target weight.

In other words, in order to hit a plateau, you have already lost some weight. Pause to reflect on the progress you have already made. Plateaus are like going through puberty: It just happens. We may not enjoy it, but we can get through it, and sometimes we can get through it with style. The following paragraphs will give you some ways of dealing with that dreaded plateau.

MUSCLE VS. FAT

An article in Everydayhealth.com [Ref-11] provides a great description of the difference between muscle and fat: "Common sense tells us a pound of muscle and a pound of fat have to weigh the same, but they do differ in density. This means if you look at five pounds of muscle and five pounds of fat side by side, the fat takes up more volume, or space, than the muscle." Because of this, when we strengthen our muscle through exercise, we will lose fat and inches. You are actually becoming thinner and more fit. Even though the scale may not reflect the fat loss, your body composition is changing for the better. This would be reflected in your measurements, photos, and the way your clothes fit. This is what people refer to as weight redistribution. There are a number of methods to track your progress. Using the scale is only one of them.

OTHER WAYS TO TRACK FAT LOSS

Take your measurements every two weeks. Make sure you measure the same exact areas at the same time of day. You can measure your neck, pecs for the men, bust and bra line for the women, the waist (at the belly button), the largest part of your hips, your biceps and your thighs.

Take photos every three to four weeks. Make sure you take them at the same time of day and in the same type of lighting. You can even wear the same clothing if you want to see how different the clothes appear on you. Keep a journal of all the activities you can do now that were difficult or impossible to do before. You can add to it whenever you notice a difference in something. It's a great way to remind yourself of the progress you have made.

Measure your body fat percentage weekly. Depending on how much you like gadgets, there are scales and electronic devices that will measure this. FYI, I found that using calipers is a pretty hard method. It is difficult to be consistent with its measurements.

Save a set of your largest clothes. It's a great motivation boost to put those old, big jeans back on and see how much smaller you are in them.

MIX IT UP

If you have been following the "Bariatric Basics" and have not shown a loss on the scale or with a reduction in measurements, here are few things you can incorporate into your routine to help kick-start your progress again.

Exercise: If you are currently walking 30 minutes per day, it's time to add some variety. Track how many steps you have been walking in 30 minutes and increase that amount by either adding more time or increasing the intensity of your walk.

Strength Training: You don't need to be a body builder, but you definitely should be toning your muscles. You can switch one of your walking days for strength training or just add it to a different time of the day. Work out with free-weights, exercise bands or your body weight to strengthen your muscles. Remember that muscle burns fat. Even if you don't see it on the scale immediately, you will in your measurements. Start by adding this one to two days per week.

Carbohydrates: Start tracking how many carbs you are eating per day. Carbohydrates turn into sugar, so this can be a hidden detriment to fat loss. The American Society for Metabolic and Bariatric Surgery (ASMBS) [Ref-12] recommends "Limiting carbohydrates to 50 grams per day or less helps avoid rebound hunger problems which can lead to weight regain."

Accountability Partner: Working with an accountability partner is fun and encouraging. Knowing you are not alone helps to keep you on track and to stay motivated. This can be with a friend, or you can hire a professional coach.

TIME TO MAKE A CHANGE

We are going to be working on an Action Goal during the next 12 weeks. An Action Goal is exactly what it sounds like: a goal which is an action, not a destination. Let's say you want to weigh 150 pounds, and today you weigh 210 pounds. Your Destination Goal is to weigh 150 pounds. You will need to lose 60 pounds to reach that long-term goal. The Action Goals are what you need to do in order to lose the 60 pounds. They are short-term goals focused on behaviors that you have control over.

Action goals are a great way to build your confidence and self-esteem. They are also the foundation to creating healthy habits that lead to long-term success. Daily, repeated and consistent behaviors create new habits. During the next 12 weeks you will be led, step by step, to create a new behavior that will become a natural part of your normal daily routine. Just like brushing your teeth.

Pretty exciting, isn't it? Ready? Let's create a new habit!

1. What is one behavior you can do (but are not doing now) on a regular basis that would make an important, positive difference in your life? Is it one of the Bariatric Basics? Is it another behavior you know you should be doing but are not doing? A clue for this behavior is that it usually has a little nagging feeling associated with it. This behavior is something you are avoiding doing regularly, even though you know it's important. Take some to think about this, and then write your answer below. (Choose a behavior other than tracking your food. You will be doing that already in this journal.)

_____

_____

_____

_____

_____

_____

2. Why aren't you doing this behavior regularly now? (Be honest with yourself.)

_____

_____

_____

_____

_____

_____

_____

_____

_____

_____

3. What can you do, right now, to incorporate this behavior into your life consistently?

_____

_____

_____

_____

_____

_____

_____

_____

_____

_____

4. How will you feel when you are doing this regularly?

_____

_____

_____

_____

_____

_____

_____

That's it. That is your Breakthrough Goal for the next 12 weeks. You are going to break through the barrier that has been holding you back. This behavior is going to become part of your everyday life. You are going to become empowered, confident and self-assured. And, that little nagging voice will finally disappear.

CREATE YOUR PLAN FOR CHANGE

Now that you know your Breakthrough Goal, it's time to create your plan for achieving it.

1. Define your goal in an easy to remember specific and measurable statement.
   Example: I will exercise for at least 20 minutes, five times per week.

_____

_____

_____

_____

2. Define the rewards for achieving this goal. What Destination Goal will be accomplished by doing this Breakthrough Goal consistently? What are the benefits for doing this? How will your life improve?

_____

_____

_____

_____

_____

_____

_____

_____

_____

_____

3. What needs to be done DAILY to achieve my WEEKLY goal? *Write out your plan for each day of the w e e k .*

MONDAY

_____

_____

_____

_____

_____

TUESDAY

_____

_____

_____

_____

_____

WEDNESDAY

_____

_____

_____

_____

_____

THURSDAY

_____
_____
_____
_____
_____
_____

FRIDAY

_____
_____
_____
_____
_____
_____

SATURDAY

_____
_____
_____
_____
_____
_____

SUNDAY

_____

_____

_____

_____

_____

_____

4. How will you deal with unexpected changes to your schedule? Write your contingency plan.

_____

_____

_____

_____

_____

_____

_____

_____

_____

_____

_____

_____

_____

_____

_____

Change begins when you take the first step.

~Beth Bianca

YOUR SUCCESS STARTS HERE

STARTING STATS	AFTER STATS
Date:	Date:
Weight:	Weight:
Chest Measurements:	Chest Measurements:
Waist Measurements:	Waist Measurements:
Hip Measurements:	Hip Measurements:

COMPLETE AND SIGN YOUR CERTIFICATE OF COMMITMENT

CERTIFICATE OF COMMITMENT

THIS CERTIFIES THAT

_____

Is Committed To Reaching This 12-Week Breakthrough Goal and Completing the Pages In This Journal Every Day.

_____
_____
_____

Date_____ Signature_____

STARTING PHOTO

Date:

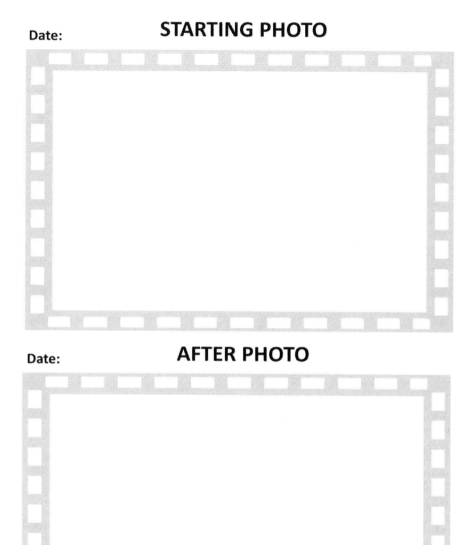

AFTER PHOTO

Date:

THE BREAKTHROUGH JOURNAL

My #1 FOCUS for today is: Exercise for 30 minutes. I am committed to doing this. No excuses!

Date: *3/01/17*

Write Your #1 Goal for the Day

Breakfast	Calories	Protein	C		
Time: *6:00 AM*					
Protein Shake with	160	25	8	1.50	2
Skim Milk	90	8	13	0	12
Totals	250	33	21	1.50	14

Record All Food Intake

Record Nutritional Information

Lunch	Calories	Protein	Carbs	Fat	Sugar
Time: *11:30 AM*					
2 Eggs Scrambled	143	12.50	0	4	0
¼ Shredded Cheese	70	8	1	4	0
¼ Cup Broccoli	15	1	2	0	1
Totals	228	21.50	3	8	1

Total Each Meal

Dinner	Calories	Protein	Carbs	Fat	Sugar
Time: *6:30 PM*					
3 oz Shredded Chicken	100	19	1	2.50	0
BBQ Sauce 2 Tbls	10	0	2	0	0
¼ Cup Broccoli	15	1	2	0	1
Totals	125	20	5	2.50	1

Snacks	Calories	Protein	Carbs	Fat	Sugar
Time: *9:00 AM Cheese Stick*	50	7	1	2.50	0
Time: *2:15 PM Chick Pattie*	140	8	15	1	1
Time: *2:15 PM Cheese*	50	7	1	2.50	
Totals	240	22	17	6	

Add All Meal Totals

Daily Totals	843	96.50	46	18	17

Water (4 ounces per square)	X X X X X X X X X X X X X X X X	
Protein (5 grams per square)	X X X X X X X X X X X X X X X X X X X	
Vitamins (1 vitamin per square)	X X	
Exercise (10 minutes per square)	X X X	

Water 4x16 =64 oz
Protein 5x19=95 g
Vitamins 1x2=2
Exercise
10x3 = 30 minutes

Mark Your Completed Bariatric Basics

Did You Accomplish Your Daily Goal?

Was my #1 FOCUS accomplished today? ☑ ☐N   My thoughts about today: Today was busy and stressful. I really didn't feel like exercising but I did it! Got my 30 minutes in. I feel so much better for following through and just getting it done. Yay Me!!

Decide and fill-in your #1 FOCUS on tomorrow's page.

I am Decisive, Determined, Disciplined and Dynamic!

Say your affirmation every time you open this page. The more you say it, the faster you'll believe it and begin to act accordingly.

There are two ways to use this coloring page.

1. As motivation for completing the Bariatric Basics every day.
   * See Below
2. Color to relieve stress from your day. Don't worry about the letters and color for pleasure at any time.

* When using the coloring page as motivation to complete the Bariatric Basics, use the completed boxes from your journal page.

Use the daily goals you have set for yourself as guidelines. The number of boxes marked as completed equal the number of letters that can be colored in on the flower.

Each flower contains the following letters:

18 Letter Ps for up to 90 grams of Protein
16 Letter Ws for up to 64 ounces of Water
06 Letter Es for up to 60 minutes of Exercise
04 Letter Vs for up to 4 Vitamins/Medications

The previous journal page shows the following information.

-WATER has 16 completed boxes. That's 64 ounces of water. All 16 Ws can be colored.

-PROTEIN has 19 completed boxes. That's 95 grams of protein. All 18 Ps can be colored.

-VITAMINS have 2 completed boxes. If you only take 2 vitamins per day, all 4 Vs can be colored. If you are supposed to take 4 vitamins, but only took 2, then only 2 Vs should be colored.

-EXERCISE has 3 completed boxes. If 30 minutes of exercise was your goal, then all 6 Es can be colored. If you only completed 20 minutes, then only 2 Es should be colored.

Completed Journal Boxes Were Used for this Example

W=Water P=Protein V=Vitamins E=Exercise

THE BREAKTHROUGH JOURNAL

First say to yourself what you would be; and then do what you have to do. ~Epictetus

My #1 FOCUS for today is:

Date:

Breakfast	Calories	Protein	Carbs	Fat	Sugar
Time:					
Totals					

Lunch	Calories	Protein	Carbs	Fat	Sugar
Time:					
Totals					

Dinner	Calories	Protein	Carbs	Fat	Sugar
Time:					
Totals					

Snacks	Calories	Protein	Carbs	Fat	Sugar
Time:					
Time:					
Time:					
Totals					

Daily Totals					

Water (4 ounces per square)																
Protein (5 grams per square)																
Vitamins (1 vitamin per square)																
Exercise (10 minutes per square)																

Was my #1 FOCUS accomplished today? Y ☐ N ☐ My thoughts about today:

Decide and fill-in your #1 FOCUS on tomorrow's page.

I am Decisive, Determined, Disciplined and Dynamic!

Day 1

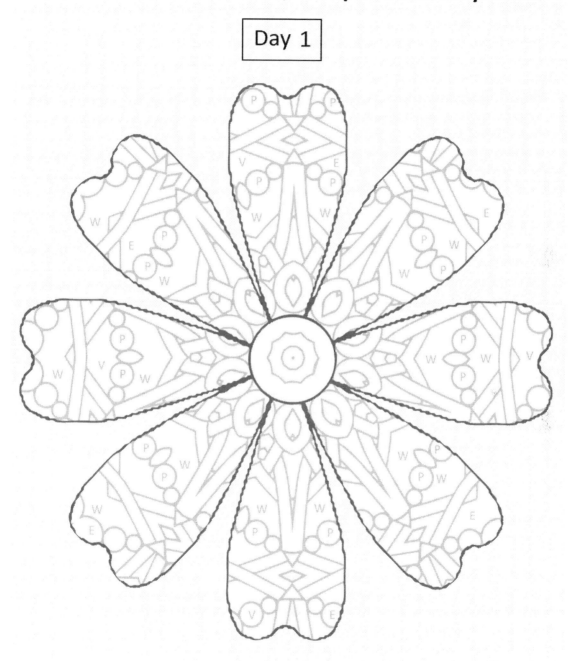

W=Water P=Protein V=Vitamins E=Exercise

THE BREAKTHROUGH JOURNAL

Your real influence is measured by your treatment of yourself. ~A. Bronson Alcott

My #1 FOCUS for today is:

Date:

Breakfast	Calories	Protein	Carbs	Fat	Sugar
Time:					
Totals					

Lunch	Calories	Protein	Carbs	Fat	Sugar
Time:					
Totals					

Dinner	Calories	Protein	Carbs	Fat	Sugar
Time:					
Totals					

Snacks	Calories	Protein	Carbs	Fat	Sugar
Time:					
Time:					
Time:					
Totals					

Daily Totals					

Water (4 ounces per square)																	
Protein (5 grams per square)																	
Vitamins (1 vitamin per square)																	
Exercise (10 minutes per square)																	

Was my #1 FOCUS accomplished today? Y ☐ N ☐ **My thoughts about today:**

Decide and fill-in your #1 FOCUS on tomorrow's page.

I am Decisive, Determined, Disciplined and Dynamic!

Day 2

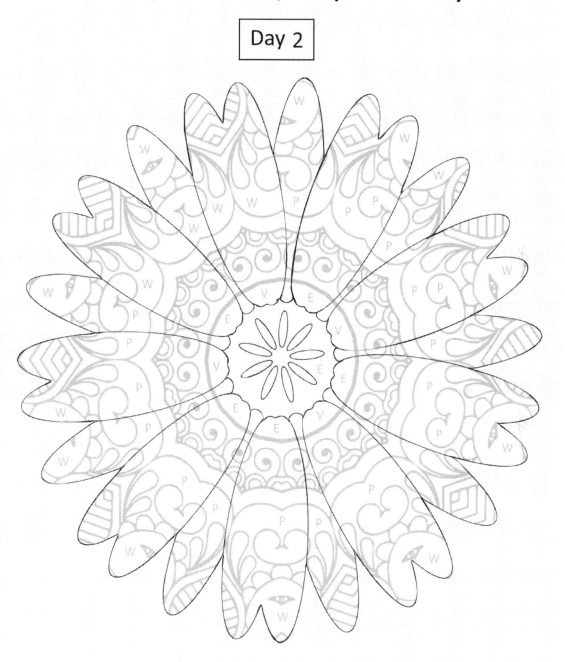

W=Water P=Protein V=Vitamins E=Exercise

THE BREAKTHROUGH JOURNAL

There is no failure except in no longer trying. ~Elbert Hubbard

My #1 FOCUS for today is:

Date:

Breakfast	Calories	Protein	Carbs	Fat	Sugar
Time:					
Totals					

Lunch	Calories	Protein	Carbs	Fat	Sugar
Time:					
Totals					

Dinner	Calories	Protein	Carbs	Fat	Sugar
Time:					
Totals					

Snacks	Calories	Protein	Carbs	Fat	Sugar
Time:					
Time:					
Time:					
Totals					

Daily Totals					

Water (4 ounces per square)																
Protein (5 grams per square)																
Vitamins (1 vitamin per square)																
Exercise (10 minutes per square)																

Was my #1 FOCUS accomplished today? Y ☐ N ☐ My thoughts about today:

Decide and fill-in your #1 FOCUS on tomorrow's page.

I am Decisive, Determined, Disciplined and Dynamic!

Day 3

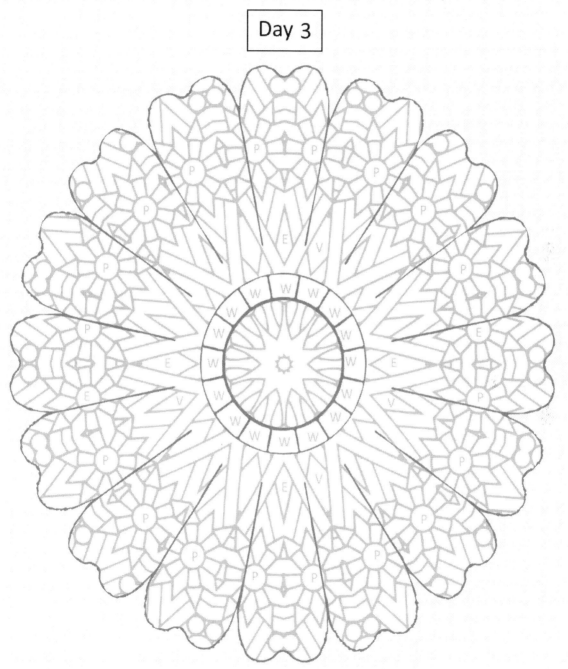

W=Water P=Protein V=Vitamins E=Exercise

THE BREAKTHROUGH JOURNAL

Take good care of your body. It's the only place you have to live. ~Jim Rohn

My #1 FOCUS for today is:

Date:

Breakfast	Calories	Protein	Carbs	Fat	Sugar
Time:					
Totals					

Lunch	Calories	Protein	Carbs	Fat	Sugar
Time:					
Totals					

Dinner	Calories	Protein	Carbs	Fat	Sugar
Time:					
Totals					

Snacks	Calories	Protein	Carbs	Fat	Sugar
Time:					
Time:					
Time:					
Totals					

Daily Totals					

Water (4 ounces per square)																
Protein (5 grams per square)																
Vitamins (1 vitamin per square)																
Exercise (10 minutes per square)																

Was my #1 FOCUS accomplished today? Y ☐ N ☐ **My thoughts about today:**

Decide and fill-in your #1 FOCUS on tomorrow's page.

I am Decisive, Determined, Disciplined and Dynamic!

Day 4

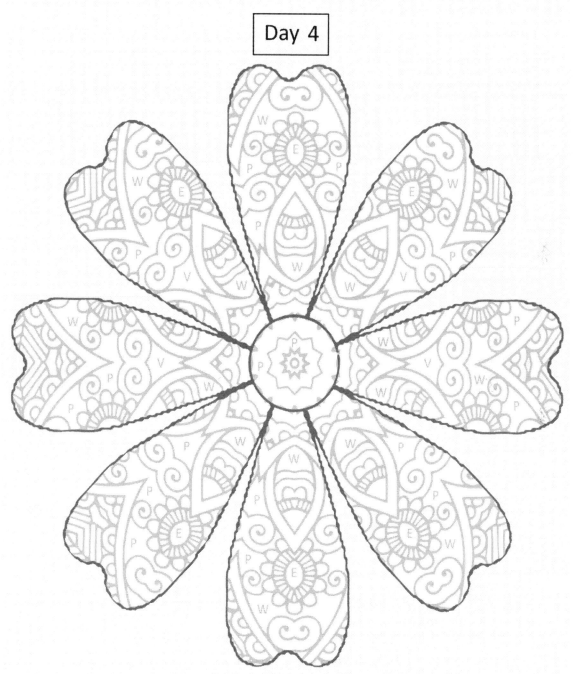

W=Water P=Protein V=Vitamins E=Exercise

THE BREAKTHROUGH JOURNAL

For changes to be of any true value, they've got to be lasting and consistent. ~Tony Robbins

My #1 FOCUS for today is:

Date:

Breakfast	Calories	Protein	Carbs	Fat	Sugar
Time:					
Totals					

Lunch	Calories	Protein	Carbs	Fat	Sugar
Time:					
Totals					

Dinner	Calories	Protein	Carbs	Fat	Sugar
Time:					
Totals					

Snacks	Calories	Protein	Carbs	Fat	Sugar
Time:					
Time:					
Time:					
Totals					

Daily Totals					

Water (4 ounces per square)									
Protein (5 grams per square)									
Vitamins (1 vitamin per square)									
Exercise (10 minutes per square)									

Was my #1 FOCUS accomplished today? Y ☐ N ☐ **My thoughts about today:**

Decide and fill-in your #1 FOCUS on tomorrow's page.

I am Decisive, Determined, Disciplined and Dynamic!

Day 5

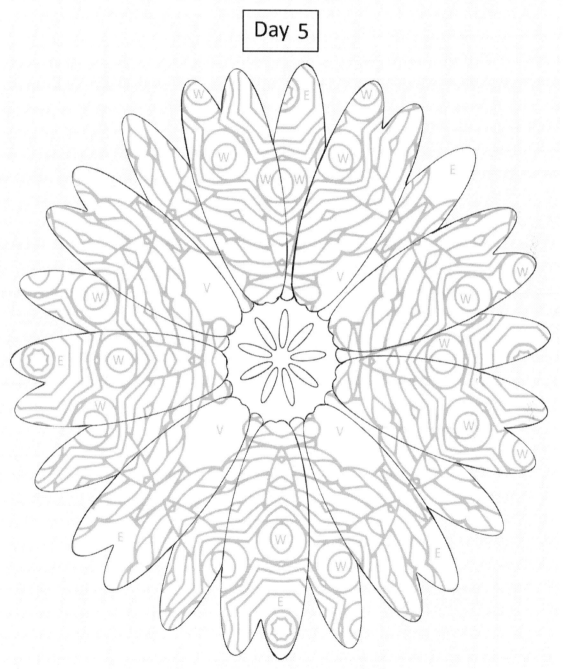

W=Water P=Protein V=Vitamins E=Exercise

THE BREAKTHROUGH JOURNAL

Successful people are simply those with successful habits. ~Brian Tracy

My #1 FOCUS for today is:

Date:

Breakfast	Calories	Protein	Carbs	Fat	Sugar
Time:					
Totals					

Lunch	Calories	Protein	Carbs	Fat	Sugar
Time:					
Totals					

Dinner	Calories	Protein	Carbs	Fat	Sugar
Time:					
Totals					

Snacks	Calories	Protein	Carbs	Fat	Sugar
Time:					
Time:					
Time:					
Totals					

Daily Totals					

Water (4 ounces per square)															
Protein (5 grams per square)															
Vitamins (1 vitamin per square)															
Exercise (10 minutes per square)															

Was my #1 FOCUS accomplished today? Y ☐ N ☐ **My thoughts about today:**

Decide and fill-in your #1 FOCUS on tomorrow's page.

I am Decisive, Determined, Disciplined and Dynamic!

Day 6

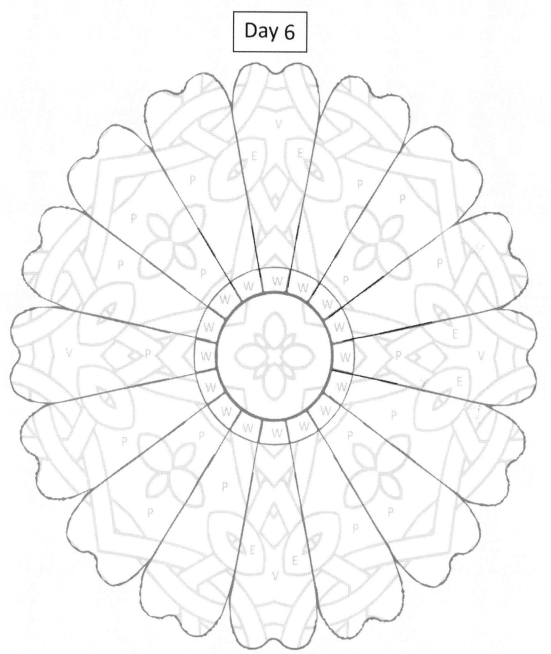

W=Water P=Protein V=Vitamins E=Exercise

THE BREAKTHROUGH JOURNAL

He who has health, has hope; and he who has hope, has everything. ~Thomas Carlyle

My #1 FOCUS for today is:

Date:

Breakfast	Calories	Protein	Carbs	Fat	Sugar
Time:					
Totals					

Lunch	Calories	Protein	Carbs	Fat	Sugar
Time:					
Totals					

Dinner	Calories	Protein	Carbs	Fat	Sugar
Time:					
Totals					

Snacks	Calories	Protein	Carbs	Fat	Sugar
Time:					
Time:					
Time:					
Totals					

Daily Totals					

Water (4 ounces per square)																
Protein (5 grams per square)																
Vitamins (1 vitamin per square)																
Exercise (10 minutes per square)																

Was my #1 FOCUS accomplished today? Y ☐ N ☐ **My thoughts about today:**

Decide and fill-in your #1 FOCUS on tomorrow's page.

THE BREAKTHROUGH JOURNAL

I am Decisive, Determined, Disciplined and Dynamic!

Day 7

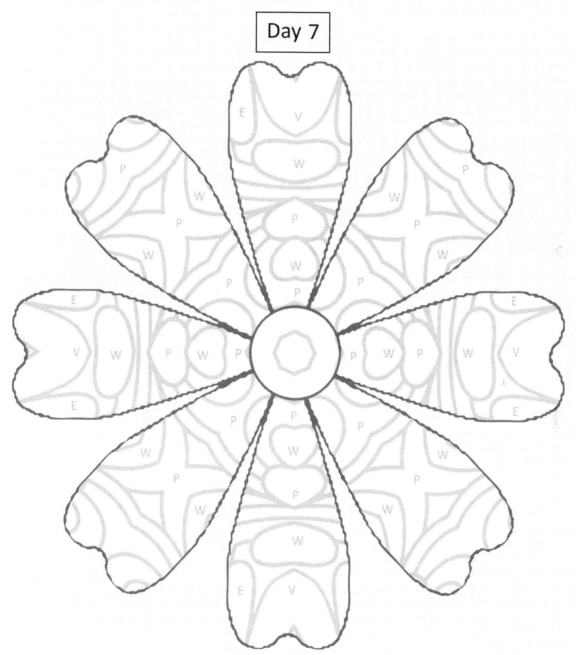

W=Water P=Protein V=Vitamins E=Exercise

WEEKLY REVIEW

Did I accomplish my goal this week?_____

What went well this week?_____

_____

_____

_____

What can be improved?_____

_____

_____

_____

My goal for the coming week is_____

_____

_____

My daily plan to accomplish this goal is_____

_____

_____

_____

_____

_____

This is the behavior I will change this week_____

_____

THOUGHTS & IDEAS

THE BREAKTHROUGH JOURNAL

Once your excuses are gone, you will simply have to settle for being awesome! ~Lorii Myers

My #1 FOCUS for today is:

Date:

Breakfast	Calories	Protein	Carbs	Fat	Sugar
Time:					
Totals					

Lunch	Calories	Protein	Carbs	Fat	Sugar
Time:					
Totals					

Dinner	Calories	Protein	Carbs	Fat	Sugar
Time:					
Totals					

Snacks	Calories	Protein	Carbs	Fat	Sugar
Time:					
Time:					
Time:					
Totals					

Daily Totals					

Water (4 ounces per square)												
Protein (5 grams per square)												
Vitamins (1 vitamin per square)												
Exercise (10 minutes per square)												

Was my #1 FOCUS accomplished today? Y ☐ N ☐ My thoughts about today:

Decide and fill-in your #1 FOCUS on tomorrow's page.

I am Decisive, Determined, Disciplined and Dynamic!

Day 8

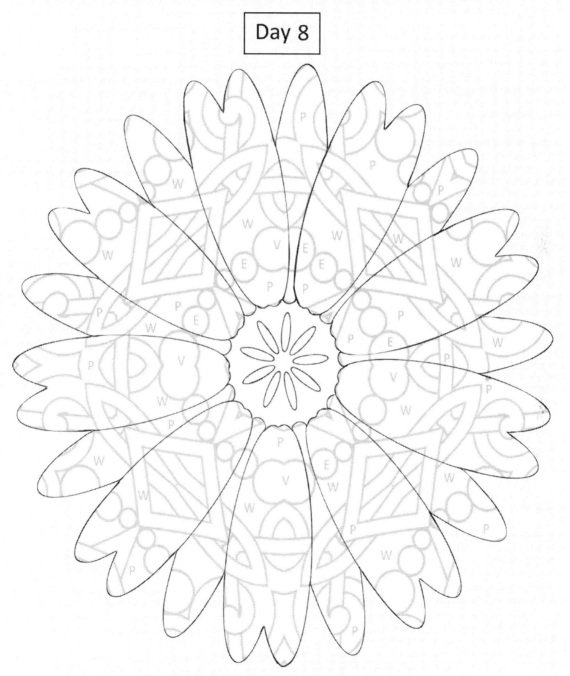

W=Water P=Protein V=Vitamins E=Exercise

THE BREAKTHROUGH JOURNAL

We become what we repeatedly do. ~Sean Covey

My #1 FOCUS for today is:

Date:

Breakfast	Calories	Protein	Carbs	Fat	Sugar
Time:					
Totals					

Lunch	Calories	Protein	Carbs	Fat	Sugar
Time:					
Totals					

Dinner	Calories	Protein	Carbs	Fat	Sugar
Time:					
Totals					

Snacks	Calories	Protein	Carbs	Fat	Sugar
Time:					
Time:					
Time:					
Totals					

Daily Totals					

Water (4 ounces per square)																			
Protein (5 grams per square)																			
Vitamins (1 vitamin per square)																			
Exercise (10 minutes per square)																			

Was my #1 FOCUS accomplished today? Y ☐ N ☐ My thoughts about today:

Decide and fill-in your #1 FOCUS on tomorrow's page.

I am Decisive, Determined, Disciplined and Dynamic!

Day 9

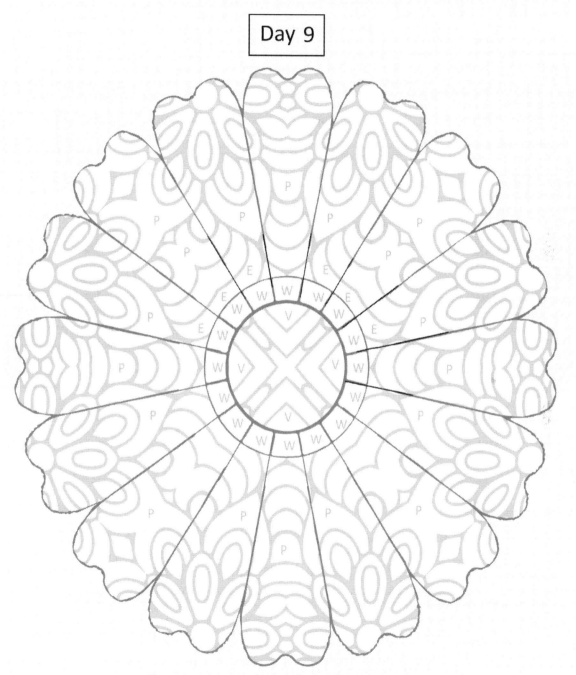

W=Water P=Protein V=Vitamins E=Exercise

THE BREAKTHROUGH JOURNAL

Fear brings failure; faith brings success. It's just that simple. ~Ernest Holmes

My #1 FOCUS for today is:

Date:

Breakfast	Calories	Protein	Carbs	Fat	Sugar
Time:					
Totals					

Lunch	Calories	Protein	Carbs	Fat	Sugar
Time:					
Totals					

Dinner	Calories	Protein	Carbs	Fat	Sugar
Time:					
Totals					

Snacks	Calories	Protein	Carbs	Fat	Sugar
Time:					
Time:					
Time:					
Totals					

Daily Totals					

Water (4 ounces per square)																		
Protein (5 grams per square)																		
Vitamins (1 vitamin per square)																		
Exercise (10 minutes per square)																		

Was my #1 FOCUS accomplished today? Y ☐ N ☐ **My thoughts about today:**

Decide and fill-in your #1 FOCUS on tomorrow's page.

THE BREAKTHROUGH JOURNAL

I am Decisive, Determined, Disciplined and Dynamic!

Day 10

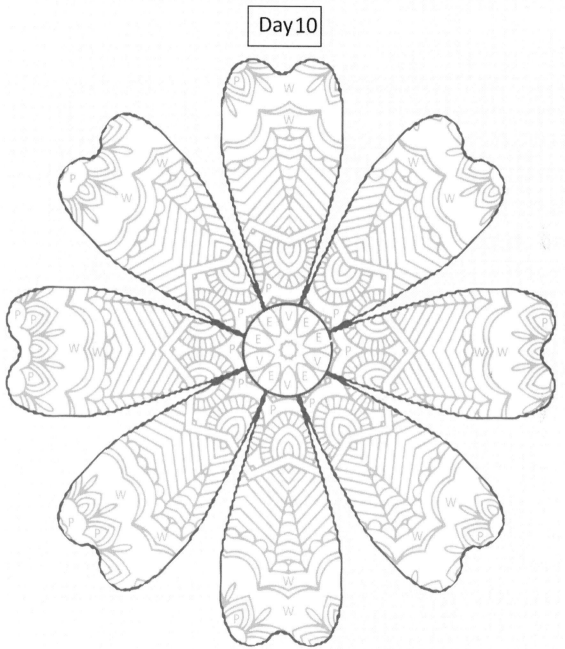

W=Water P=Protein V=Vitamins E=Exercise

THE BREAKTHROUGH JOURNAL

A man is but the product of his thoughts what he thinks, he becomes. ~Mahatma Gandhi

My #1 FOCUS for today is:

Date:

Breakfast	Calories	Protein	Carbs	Fat	Sugar
Time:					
Totals					

Lunch	Calories	Protein	Carbs	Fat	Sugar
Time:					
Totals					

Dinner	Calories	Protein	Carbs	Fat	Sugar
Time:					
Totals					

Snacks	Calories	Protein	Carbs	Fat	Sugar
Time:					
Time:					
Time:					
Totals					

Daily Totals					

Water (4 ounces per square)																	
Protein (5 grams per square)																	
Vitamins (1 vitamin per square)																	
Exercise (10 minutes per square)																	

Was my #1 FOCUS accomplished today? Y ☐ N ☐ My thoughts about today:

Decide and fill-in your #1 FOCUS on tomorrow's page.

THE BREAKTHROUGH JOURNAL

I am Decisive, Determined, Disciplined and Dynamic!

Day 11

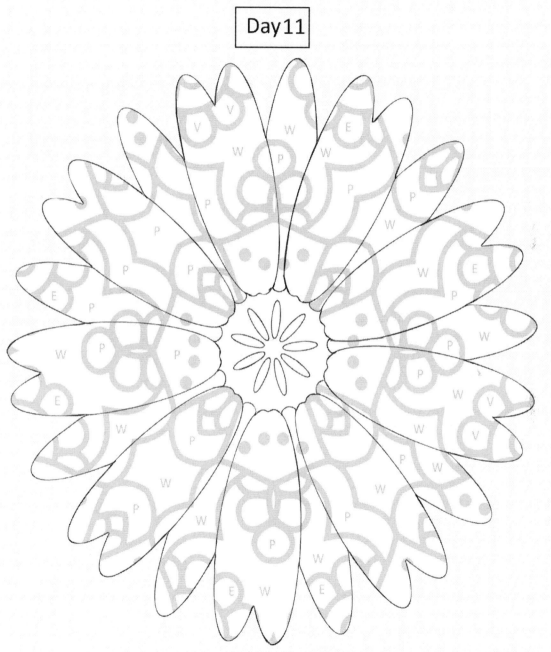

W=Water P=Protein V=Vitamins E=Exercise

THE BREAKTHROUGH JOURNAL

Positive thinking will let you do everything better than negative thinking will. ~Zig Ziglar

My #1 FOCUS for today is:

Date:

Breakfast	Calories	Protein	Carbs	Fat	Sugar
Time:					
Totals					

Lunch	Calories	Protein	Carbs	Fat	Sugar
Time:					
Totals					

Dinner	Calories	Protein	Carbs	Fat	Sugar
Time:					
Totals					

Snacks	Calories	Protein	Carbs	Fat	Sugar
Time:					
Time:					
Time:					
Totals					

Daily Totals					

Water (4 ounces per square)																
Protein (5 grams per square)																
Vitamins (1 vitamin per square)																
Exercise (10 minutes per square)																

Was my #1 FOCUS accomplished today? Y ☐ N ☐ My thoughts about today:

Decide and fill-in your #1 FOCUS on tomorrow's page.

I am Decisive, Determined, Disciplined and Dynamic!

Day 12

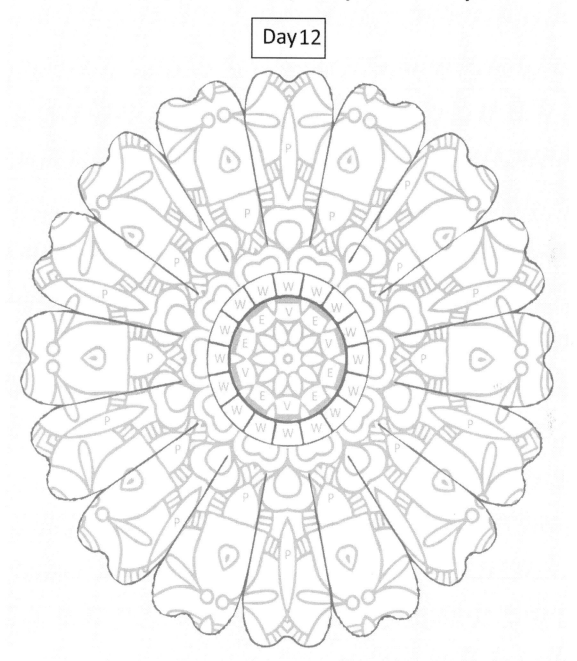

W=Water P=Protein V=Vitamins E=Exercise

THE BREAKTHROUGH JOURNAL

Remember, today is the tomorrow you worried about yesterday. ~Dale Carnegie

My #1 FOCUS for today is:

Date:

Breakfast	Calories	Protein	Carbs	Fat	Sugar
Time:					
Totals					

Lunch	Calories	Protein	Carbs	Fat	Sugar
Time:					
Totals					

Dinner	Calories	Protein	Carbs	Fat	Sugar
Time:					
Totals					

Snacks	Calories	Protein	Carbs	Fat	Sugar
Time:					
Time:					
Time:					
Totals					

Daily Totals					

Water (4 ounces per square)																		
Protein (5 grams per square)																		
Vitamins (1 vitamin per square)																		
Exercise (10 minutes per square)																		

Was my #1 FOCUS accomplished today? Y ☐ N ☐ My thoughts about today:

Decide and fill-in your #1 FOCUS on tomorrow's page.

I am Decisive, Determined, Disciplined and Dynamic!

Day 13

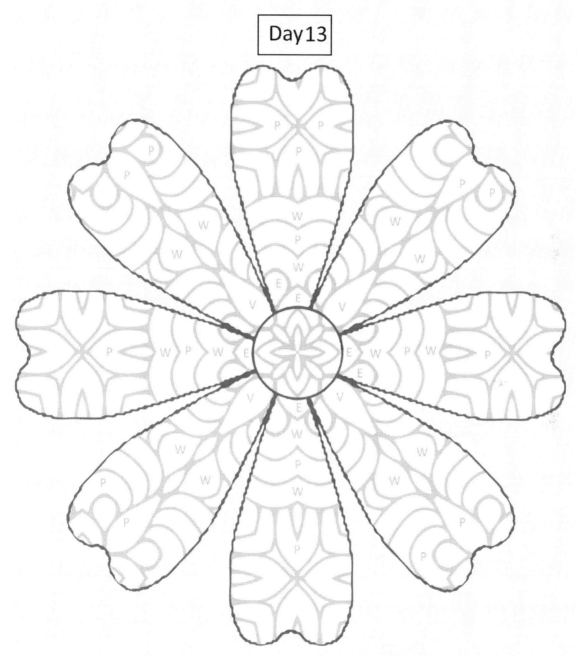

W=Water P=Protein V=Vitamins E=Exercise

THE BREAKTHROUGH JOURNAL

All the art of living lies in a fine mingling of letting go and holding on. ~Henry Ellis

My #1 FOCUS for today is:

Date:

Breakfast	Calories	Protein	Carbs	Fat	Sugar
Time:					
Totals					

Lunch	Calories	Protein	Carbs	Fat	Sugar
Time:					
Totals					

Dinner	Calories	Protein	Carbs	Fat	Sugar
Time:					
Totals					

Snacks	Calories	Protein	Carbs	Fat	Sugar
Time:					
Time:					
Time:					
Totals					

Daily Totals					

Water (4 ounces per square)																	
Protein (5 grams per square)																	
Vitamins (1 vitamin per square)																	
Exercise (10 minutes per square)																	

Was my #1 FOCUS accomplished today? Y ☐ N ☐ **My thoughts about today:**

Decide and fill-in your #1 FOCUS on tomorrow's page.

I am Decisive, Determined, Disciplined and Dynamic!

Day 14

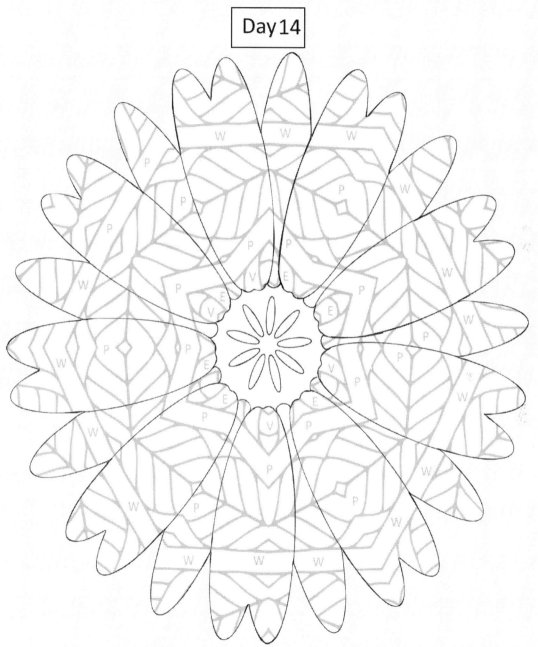

W=Water P=Protein V=Vitamins E=Exercise

WEEKLY REVIEW

Did I accomplish my goal this week?_____

What went well this week?_____

_____

_____

_____

What can be improved?_____

_____

_____

_____

My goal for the coming week is_____

_____

_____

My daily plan to accomplish this goal is_____

_____

_____

_____

_____

_____

This is the behavior I will change this week_____

_____

THOUGHTS & IDEAS

THE BREAKTHROUGH JOURNAL

Once you figure out what you want in life – expect nothing less. ~Lorii Meyers

My #1 FOCUS for today is:

Date:

Breakfast	Calories	Protein	Carbs	Fat	Sugar
Time:					
Totals					

Lunch	Calories	Protein	Carbs	Fat	Sugar
Time:					
Totals					

Dinner	Calories	Protein	Carbs	Fat	Sugar
Time:					
Totals					

Snacks	Calories	Protein	Carbs	Fat	Sugar
Time:					
Time:					
Time:					
Totals					

Daily Totals					

Water (4 ounces per square)																
Protein (5 grams per square)																
Vitamins (1 vitamin per square)																
Exercise (10 minutes per square)																

Was my #1 FOCUS accomplished today? Y ☐ N ☐ My thoughts about today:

Decide and fill-in your #1 FOCUS on tomorrow's page.

THE BREAKTHROUGH JOURNAL
I am Decisive, Determined, Disciplined and Dynamic!

Day 15

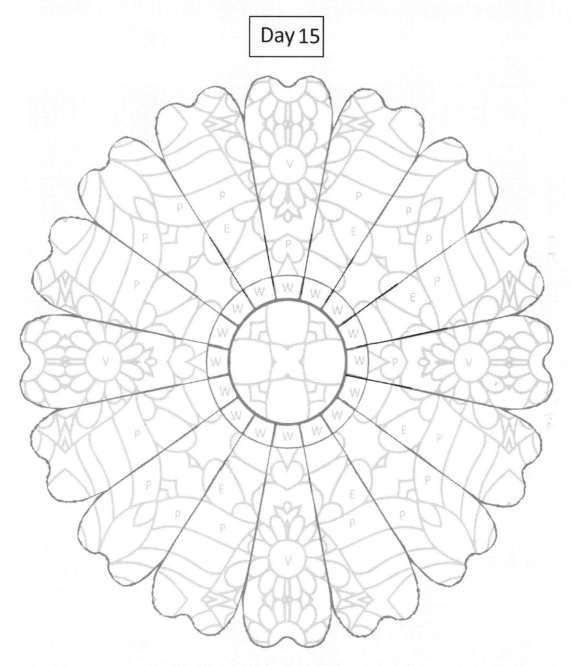

W=Water P=Protein V=Vitamins E=Exercise

THE BREAKTHROUGH JOURNAL

If you don't run your own life, somebody else will. ~John Atkinson

My #1 FOCUS for today is:

Date:

Breakfast	Calories	Protein	Carbs	Fat	Sugar
Time:					
Totals					

Lunch	Calories	Protein	Carbs	Fat	Sugar
Time:					
Totals					

Dinner	Calories	Protein	Carbs	Fat	Sugar
Time:					
Totals					

Snacks	Calories	Protein	Carbs	Fat	Sugar
Time:					
Time:					
Time:					
Totals					

Daily Totals					

Water (4 ounces per square)																	
Protein (5 grams per square)																	
Vitamins (1 vitamin per square)																	
Exercise (10 minutes per square)																	

Was my #1 FOCUS accomplished today? Y ☐ N ☐ **My thoughts about today:**

Decide and fill-in your #1 FOCUS on tomorrow's page.

I am Decisive, Determined, Disciplined and Dynamic!

Day 16

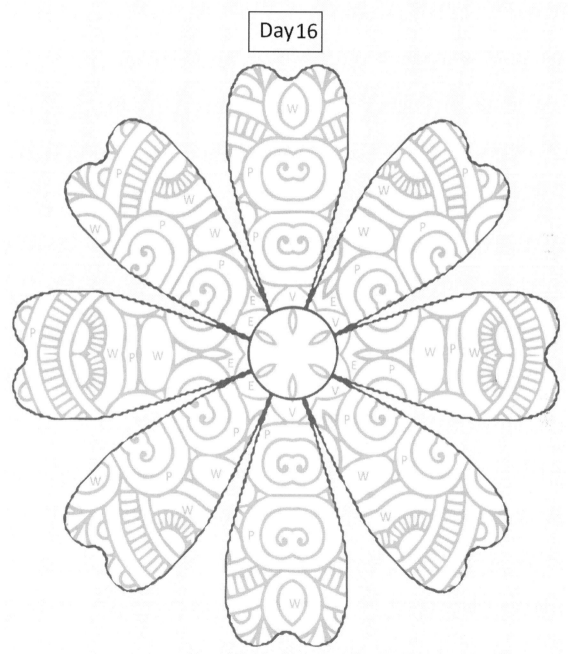

W=Water P=Protein V=Vitamins E=Exercise

THE BREAKTHROUGH JOURNAL

Believe you can and you're halfway there. ~Theodore Roosevelt

My #1 FOCUS for today is:

Date:

Breakfast	Calories	Protein	Carbs	Fat	Sugar
Time:					
Totals					

Lunch	Calories	Protein	Carbs	Fat	Sugar
Time:					
Totals					

Dinner	Calories	Protein	Carbs	Fat	Sugar
Time:					
Totals					

Snacks	Calories	Protein	Carbs	Fat	Sugar
Time:					
Time:					
Time:					
Totals					

Daily Totals					

Water (4 ounces per square)																
Protein (5 grams per square)																
Vitamins (1 vitamin per square)																
Exercise (10 minutes per square)																

Was my #1 FOCUS accomplished today? Y ☐ N ☐ **My thoughts about today:**

Decide and fill-in your #1 FOCUS on tomorrow's page.

I am Decisive, Determined, Disciplined and Dynamic!

Day 17

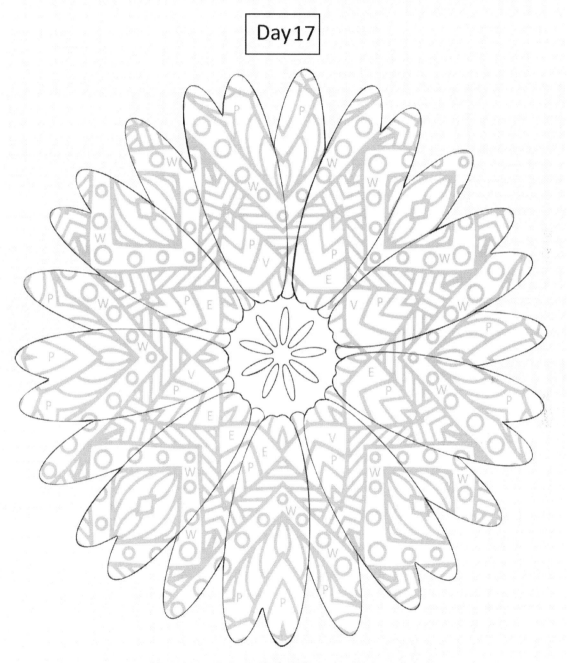

W=Water P=Protein V=Vitamins E=Exercise

THE BREAKTHROUGH JOURNAL

Happiness is not something you postpone for the future; it is something you design for the present. ~Jim Rohn

My #1 FOCUS for today is:

Date:

Breakfast	Calories	Protein	Carbs	Fat	Sugar
Time:					
Totals					

Lunch	Calories	Protein	Carbs	Fat	Sugar
Time:					
Totals					

Dinner	Calories	Protein	Carbs	Fat	Sugar
Time:					
Totals					

Snacks	Calories	Protein	Carbs	Fat	Sugar
Time:					
Time:					
Time:					
Totals					

Daily Totals					

Water (4 ounces per square)																
Protein (5 grams per square)																
Vitamins (1 vitamin per square)																
Exercise (10 minutes per square)																

Was my #1 FOCUS accomplished today? Y ☐ N ☐ **My thoughts about today:**

Decide and fill-in your #1 FOCUS on tomorrow's page.

I am Decisive, Determined, Disciplined and Dynamic!

Day 18

W=Water P=Protein V=Vitamins E=Exercise

THE BREAKTHROUGH JOURNAL

Never say anything about yourself you do not want to come true. ~Brian Tracy

My #1 FOCUS for today is:

Date:

Breakfast	Calories	Protein	Carbs	Fat	Sugar
Time:					
Totals					

Lunch	Calories	Protein	Carbs	Fat	Sugar
Time:					
Totals					

Dinner	Calories	Protein	Carbs	Fat	Sugar
Time:					
Totals					

Snacks	Calories	Protein	Carbs	Fat	Sugar
Time:					
Time:					
Time:					
Totals					

Daily Totals					

Water (4 ounces per square)																
Protein (5 grams per square)																
Vitamins (1 vitamin per square)																
Exercise (10 minutes per square)																

Was my #1 FOCUS accomplished today? Y ☐ N ☐ **My thoughts about today:**

Decide and fill-in your #1 FOCUS on tomorrow's page.

I am Decisive, Determined, Disciplined and Dynamic!

Day 19

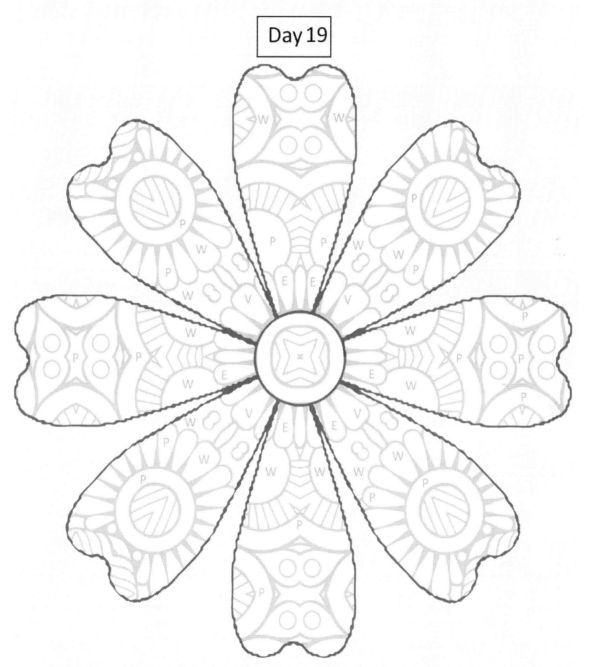

W=Water P=Protein V=Vitamins E=Exercise

THE BREAKTHROUGH JOURNAL

If you do not conquer self, you will be conquered by self. ~Napoleon Hill

My #1 FOCUS for today is:

Date:

Breakfast	Calories	Protein	Carbs	Fat	Sugar
Time:					
Totals					

Lunch	Calories	Protein	Carbs	Fat	Sugar
Time:					
Totals					

Dinner	Calories	Protein	Carbs	Fat	Sugar
Time:					
Totals					

Snacks	Calories	Protein	Carbs	Fat	Sugar
Time:					
Time:					
Time:					
Totals					

Daily Totals					

Water (4 ounces per square)															
Protein (5 grams per square)															
Vitamins (1 vitamin per square)															
Exercise (10 minutes per square)															

Was my #1 FOCUS accomplished today? Y ☐ N ☐ **My thoughts about today:**

Decide and fill-in your #1 FOCUS on tomorrow's page.

I am Decisive, Determined, Disciplined and Dynamic!

Day 20

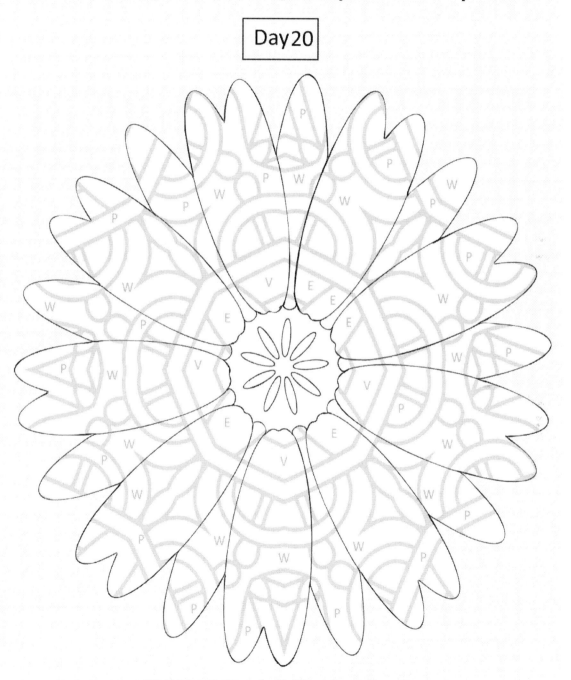

W=Water P=Protein V=Vitamins E=Exercise

THE BREAKTHROUGH JOURNAL

The mind that is anxious about future events is miserable. ~Seneca

My #1 FOCUS for today is:

Date:

Breakfast	Calories	Protein	Carbs	Fat	Sugar
Time:					
Totals					

Lunch	Calories	Protein	Carbs	Fat	Sugar
Time:					
Totals					

Dinner	Calories	Protein	Carbs	Fat	Sugar
Time:					
Totals					

Snacks	Calories	Protein	Carbs	Fat	Sugar
Time:					
Time:					
Time:					
Totals					

Daily Totals					

Water (4 ounces per square)																	
Protein (5 grams per square)																	
Vitamins (1 vitamin per square)																	
Exercise (10 minutes per square)																	

Was my #1 FOCUS accomplished today? Y ☐ N ☐ **My thoughts about today:**

Decide and fill-in your #1 FOCUS on tomorrow's page.

THE BREAKTHROUGH JOURNAL

I am Decisive, Determined, Disciplined and Dynamic!

Day 21

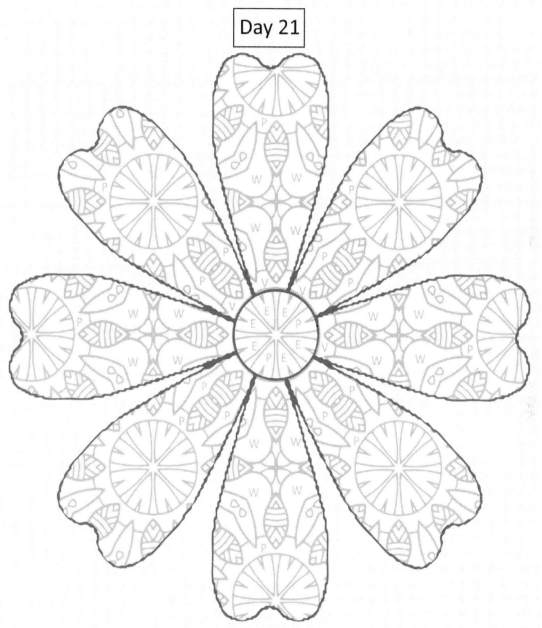

W=Water P=Protein V=Vitamins E=Exercise

WEEKLY REVIEW

Did I accomplish my goal this week?_____

What went well this week?_____

_____

_____

_____

What can be improved?_____

_____

_____

_____

My goal for the coming week is_____

_____

_____

My daily plan to accomplish this goal is_____

_____

_____

_____

_____

_____

_____

This is the behavior I will change this week_____

_____

THOUGHTS & IDEAS

THE BREAKTHROUGH JOURNAL

If we wait for the moment when everything, absolutely everything is ready, we shall never begin. ~Ivan Turgenev

My #1 FOCUS for today is:

Date:

Breakfast	Calories	Protein	Carbs	Fat	Sugar
Time:					
Totals					

Lunch	Calories	Protein	Carbs	Fat	Sugar
Time:					
Totals					

Dinner	Calories	Protein	Carbs	Fat	Sugar
Time:					
Totals					

Snacks	Calories	Protein	Carbs	Fat	Sugar
Time:					
Time:					
Time:					
Totals					

Daily Totals					

Water (4 ounces per square)																
Protein (5 grams per square)																
Vitamins (1 vitamin per square)																
Exercise (10 minutes per square)																

Was my #1 FOCUS accomplished today? Y ☐ N ☐ **My thoughts about today:**

Decide and fill-in your #1 FOCUS on tomorrow's page.

I am Decisive, Determined, Disciplined and Dynamic!

Day 22

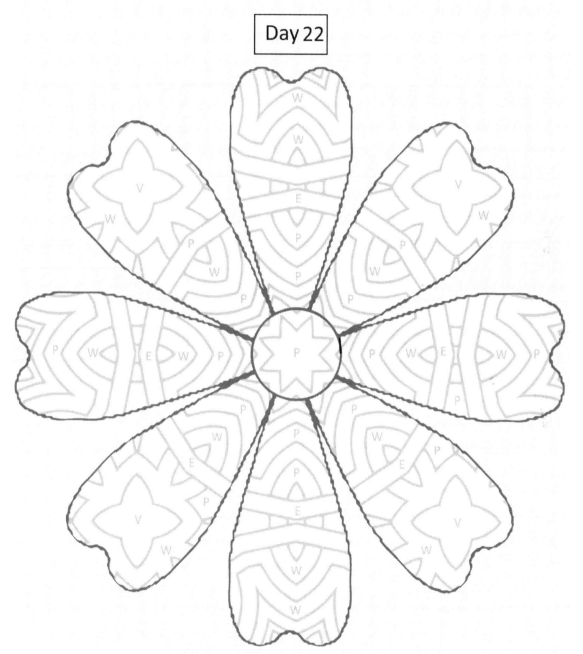

W=Water P=Protein V=Vitamins E=Exercise

THE BREAKTHROUGH JOURNAL

There's always a way - if you're committed. ~Tony Robbins

My #1 FOCUS for today is:

Date:

Breakfast	Calories	Protein	Carbs	Fat	Sugar
Time:					
Totals					

Lunch	Calories	Protein	Carbs	Fat	Sugar
Time:					
Totals					

Dinner	Calories	Protein	Carbs	Fat	Sugar
Time:					
Totals					

Snacks	Calories	Protein	Carbs	Fat	Sugar
Time:					
Time:					
Time:					
Totals					

Daily Totals					

Water (4 ounces per square)															
Protein (5 grams per square)															
Vitamins (1 vitamin per square)															
Exercise (10 minutes per square)															

Was my #1 FOCUS accomplished today? Y ☐ N ☐ **My thoughts about today:**

Decide and fill-in your #1 FOCUS on tomorrow's page.

THE BREAKTHROUGH JOURNAL
I am Decisive, Determined, Disciplined and Dynamic!

Day 23

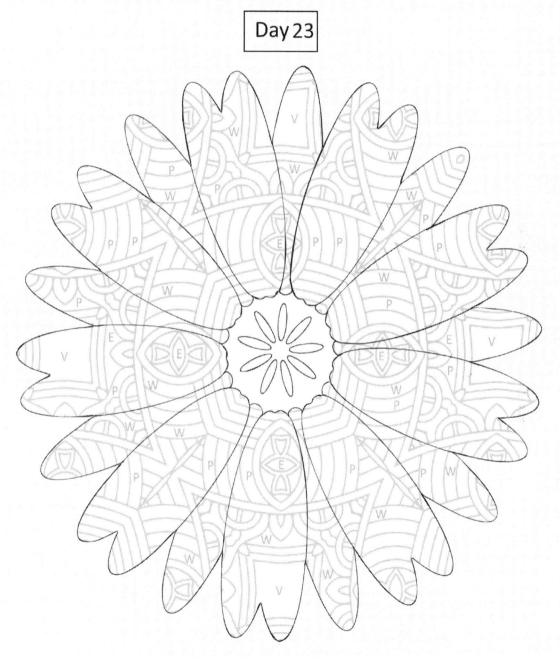

W=Water P=Protein V=Vitamins E=Exercise

THE BREAKTHROUGH JOURNAL

Well done is better than well said. ~Benjamin Franklin

My #1 FOCUS for today is:

Date:

Breakfast	Calories	Protein	Carbs	Fat	Sugar
Time:					
Totals					

Lunch	Calories	Protein	Carbs	Fat	Sugar
Time:					
Totals					

Dinner	Calories	Protein	Carbs	Fat	Sugar
Time:					
Totals					

Snacks	Calories	Protein	Carbs	Fat	Sugar
Time:					
Time:					
Time:					
Totals					

Daily Totals					

Water (4 ounces per square)																			
Protein (5 grams per square)																			
Vitamins (1 vitamin per square)																			
Exercise (10 minutes per square)																			

Was my #1 FOCUS accomplished today? Y ☐ N ☐ **My thoughts about today:**

Decide and fill-in your #1 FOCUS on tomorrow's page.

THE BREAKTHROUGH JOURNAL
I am Decisive, Determined, Disciplined and Dynamic!

Day 24

W=Water P=Protein V=Vitamins E=Exercise

THE BREAKTHROUGH JOURNAL

You can't do anything about the length of your life, but you can do something about its width and depth. ~Shira Tehrani

My #1 FOCUS for today is:

Date:

Breakfast	Calories	Protein	Carbs	Fat	Sugar
Time:					
Totals					

Lunch	Calories	Protein	Carbs	Fat	Sugar
Time:					
Totals					

Dinner	Calories	Protein	Carbs	Fat	Sugar
Time:					
Totals					

Snacks	Calories	Protein	Carbs	Fat	Sugar
Time:					
Time:					
Time:					
Totals					

Daily Totals					

Water (4 ounces per square)																	
Protein (5 grams per square)																	
Vitamins (1 vitamin per square)																	
Exercise (10 minutes per square)																	

Was my #1 FOCUS accomplished today? Y ☐ N ☐ My thoughts about today:

Decide and fill-in your #1 FOCUS on tomorrow's page.

I am Decisive, Determined, Disciplined and Dynamic!

Day 25

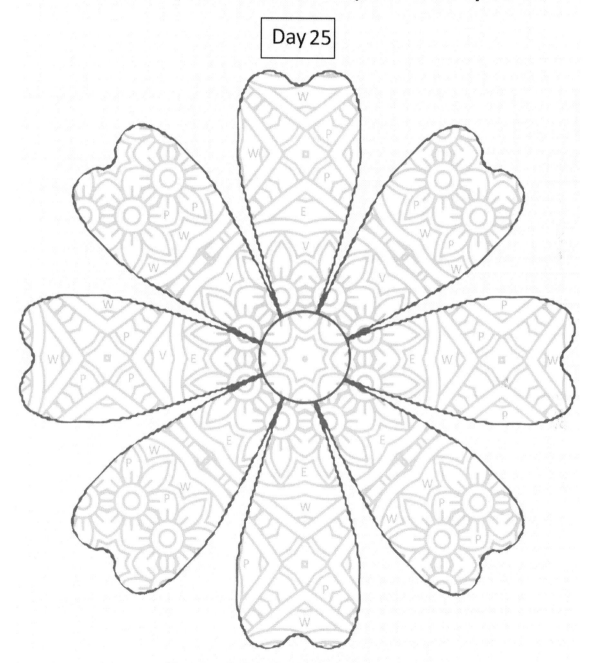

W=Water P=Protein V=Vitamins E=Exercise

THE BREAKTHROUGH JOURNAL

Every day do something that will inch you closer to a better tomorrow. ~Doug Firebaugh

My #1 FOCUS for today is:

Date:

Breakfast	Calories	Protein	Carbs	Fat	Sugar
Time:					
Totals					

Lunch	Calories	Protein	Carbs	Fat	Sugar
Time:					
Totals					

Dinner	Calories	Protein	Carbs	Fat	Sugar
Time:					
Totals					

Snacks	Calories	Protein	Carbs	Fat	Sugar
Time:					
Time:					
Time:					
Totals					

Daily Totals					

Water (4 ounces per square)																
Protein (5 grams per square)																
Vitamins (1 vitamin per square)																
Exercise (10 minutes per square)																

Was my #1 FOCUS accomplished today? Y ☐ N ☐ My thoughts about today:

Decide and fill-in your #1 FOCUS on tomorrow's page.

I am Decisive, Determined, Disciplined and Dynamic!

Day 26

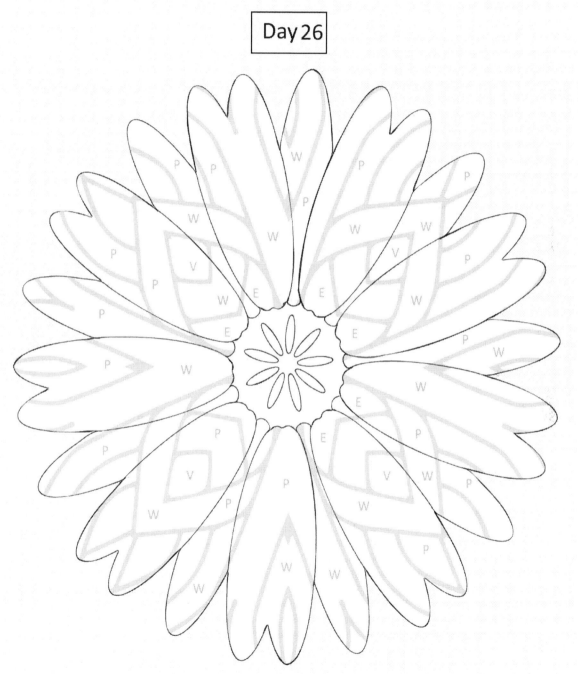

W=Water P=Protein V=Vitamins E=Exercise

THE BREAKTHROUGH JOURNAL

What we dwell on is who we become. ~Oprah Winfrey

My #1 FOCUS for today is:

Date:

Breakfast	Calories	Protein	Carbs	Fat	Sugar
Time:					
Totals					

Lunch	Calories	Protein	Carbs	Fat	Sugar
Time:					
Totals					

Dinner	Calories	Protein	Carbs	Fat	Sugar
Time:					
Totals					

Snacks	Calories	Protein	Carbs	Fat	Sugar
Time:					
Time:					
Time:					
Totals					

Daily Totals					

Water (4 ounces per square)																
Protein (5 grams per square)																
Vitamins (1 vitamin per square)																
Exercise (10 minutes per square)																

Was my #1 FOCUS accomplished today? Y ☐ N ☐ My thoughts about today:

Decide and fill-in your #1 FOCUS on tomorrow's page.

I am Decisive, Determined, Disciplined and Dynamic!

Day 27

W=Water P=Protein V=Vitamins E=Exercise

THE BREAKTHROUGH JOURNAL

Willpower is the unflinching purpose to see a task through to completion. ~Jerry Bruckner

My #1 FOCUS for today is:

Date:

Breakfast	Calories	Protein	Carbs	Fat	Sugar
Time:					
Totals					

Lunch	Calories	Protein	Carbs	Fat	Sugar
Time:					
Totals					

Dinner	Calories	Protein	Carbs	Fat	Sugar
Time:					
Totals					

Snacks	Calories	Protein	Carbs	Fat	Sugar
Time:					
Time:					
Time:					
Totals					

Daily Totals					

Water (4 ounces per square)																		
Protein (5 grams per square)																		
Vitamins (1 vitamin per square)																		
Exercise (10 minutes per square)																		

Was my #1 FOCUS accomplished today? Y ☐ N ☐   **My thoughts about today:**

Decide and fill-in your #1 FOCUS on tomorrow's page.

THE BREAKTHROUGH JOURNAL

I am Decisive, Determined, Disciplined and Dynamic!

Day 28

W=Water P=Protein V=Vitamins E=Exercise

WEEKLY REVIEW

Did I accomplish my goal this week?_____

What went well this week?_____

_____

_____

_____

What can be improved?_____

_____

_____

_____

My goal for the coming week is_____

_____

_____

My daily plan to accomplish this goal is_____

_____

_____

_____

_____

_____

_____

This is the behavior I will change this week_____

MONTHLY REVIEW

Date:_____

Weight:_____

Bust Measurement:_____

Waist Measurement:_____

Hips Measurement:_____

My major accomplishments during the last 4 weeks were_____

_____

_____

_____

What do I need to improve during the next 4 weeks?_____

_____

_____

My goal for the next 4 weeks is_____

_____

_____

My weekly plan to accomplish this goal during the next 4 weeks is_____

_____

_____

_____

_____

THE BREAKTHROUGH JOURNAL

Think big thoughts that give you strength and make you resilient. ~Jerry Bruckner

My #1 FOCUS for today is:

Date:

Breakfast	Calories	Protein	Carbs	Fat	Sugar
Time:					
Totals					

Lunch	Calories	Protein	Carbs	Fat	Sugar
Time:					
Totals					

Dinner	Calories	Protein	Carbs	Fat	Sugar
Time:					
Totals					

Snacks	Calories	Protein	Carbs	Fat	Sugar
Time:					
Time:					
Time:					
Totals					

Daily Totals					

Water (4 ounces per square)																		
Protein (5 grams per square)																		
Vitamins (1 vitamin per square)																		
Exercise (10 minutes per square)																		

Was my #1 FOCUS accomplished today? Y ☐ N ☐ **My thoughts about today:**

Decide and fill-in your #1 FOCUS on tomorrow's page.

I am Decisive, Determined, Disciplined and Dynamic!

Day 29

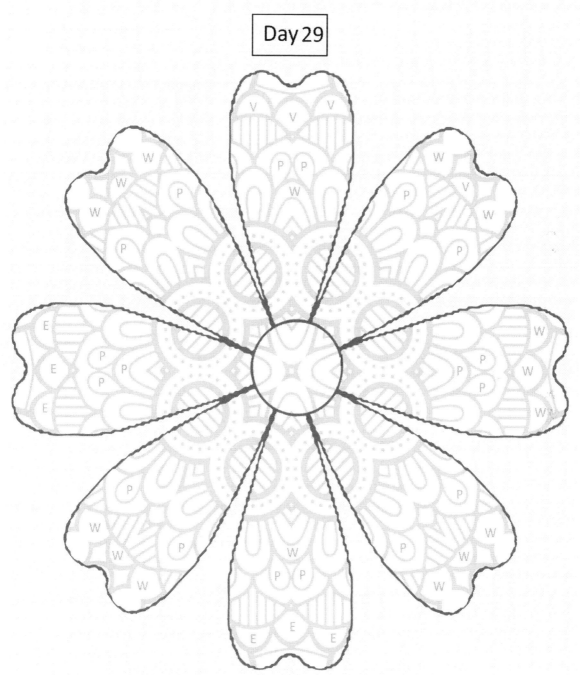

W=Water P=Protein V=Vitamins E=Exercise

THE BREAKTHROUGH JOURNAL

When you know what's important, it's a lot easier to ignore what's not. ~Marie Forleo

My #1 FOCUS for today is:

Date:

Breakfast	Calories	Protein	Carbs	Fat	Sugar
Time:					
Totals					

Lunch	Calories	Protein	Carbs	Fat	Sugar
Time:					
Totals					

Dinner	Calories	Protein	Carbs	Fat	Sugar
Time:					
Totals					

Snacks	Calories	Protein	Carbs	Fat	Sugar
Time:					
Time:					
Time:					
Totals					

Daily Totals					

Water (4 ounces per square)															
Protein (5 grams per square)															
Vitamins (1 vitamin per square)															
Exercise (10 minutes per square)															

Was my #1 FOCUS accomplished today? Y ☐ N ☐ **My thoughts about today:**

Decide and fill-in your #1 FOCUS on tomorrow's page.

THE BREAKTHROUGH JOURNAL

I am Decisive, Determined, Disciplined and Dynamic!

Day 30

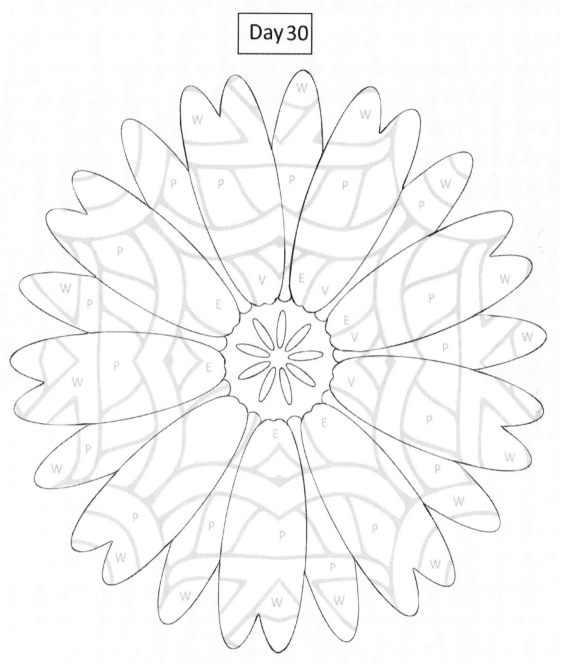

W=Water P=Protein V=Vitamins E=Exercise

THE BREAKTHROUGH JOURNAL

Belief creates the actual fact. ~William James

My #1 FOCUS for today is:

Date:

Breakfast	Calories	Protein	Carbs	Fat	Sugar
Time:					
Totals					

Lunch	Calories	Protein	Carbs	Fat	Sugar
Time:					
Totals					

Dinner	Calories	Protein	Carbs	Fat	Sugar
Time:					
Totals					

Snacks	Calories	Protein	Carbs	Fat	Sugar
Time:					
Time:					
Time:					
Totals					

Daily Totals					

Water (4 ounces per square)																		
Protein (5 grams per square)																		
Vitamins (1 vitamin per square)																		
Exercise (10 minutes per square)																		

Was my #1 FOCUS accomplished today? Y ☐ N ☐ **My thoughts about today:**

Decide and fill-in your #1 FOCUS on tomorrow's page.

I am Decisive, Determined, Disciplined and Dynamic!

Day 31

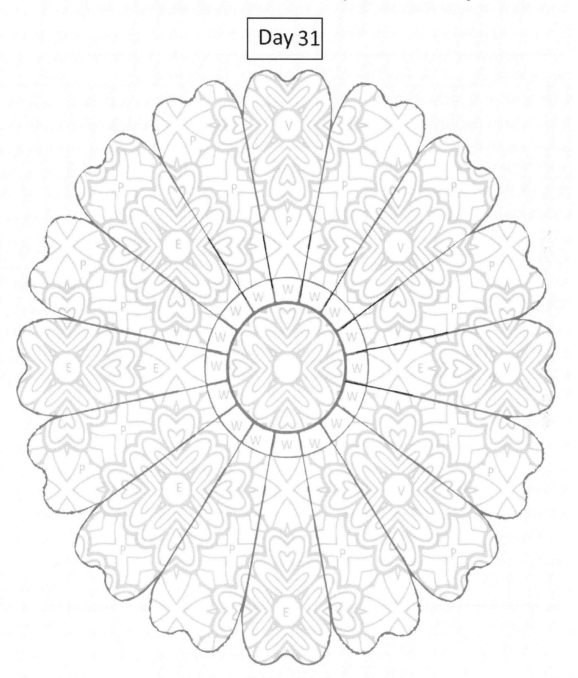

W=Water P=Protein V=Vitamins E=Exercise

THE BREAKTHROUGH JOURNAL

The only person you are destined to become is the person you decide to be. ~Ralph Waldo Emerson

My #1 FOCUS for today is:

Date:

Breakfast	Calories	Protein	Carbs	Fat	Sugar
Time:					
Totals					

Lunch	Calories	Protein	Carbs	Fat	Sugar
Time:					
Totals					

Dinner	Calories	Protein	Carbs	Fat	Sugar
Time:					
Totals					

Snacks	Calories	Protein	Carbs	Fat	Sugar
Time:					
Time:					
Time:					
Totals					

Daily Totals					

Water (4 ounces per square)																	
Protein (5 grams per square)																	
Vitamins (1 vitamin per square)																	
Exercise (10 minutes per square)																	

Was my #1 FOCUS accomplished today? Y ☐ N ☐   My thoughts about today:

Decide and fill-in your #1 FOCUS on tomorrow's page.

THE BREAKTHROUGH JOURNAL

I am Decisive, Determined, Disciplined and Dynamic!

Day 32

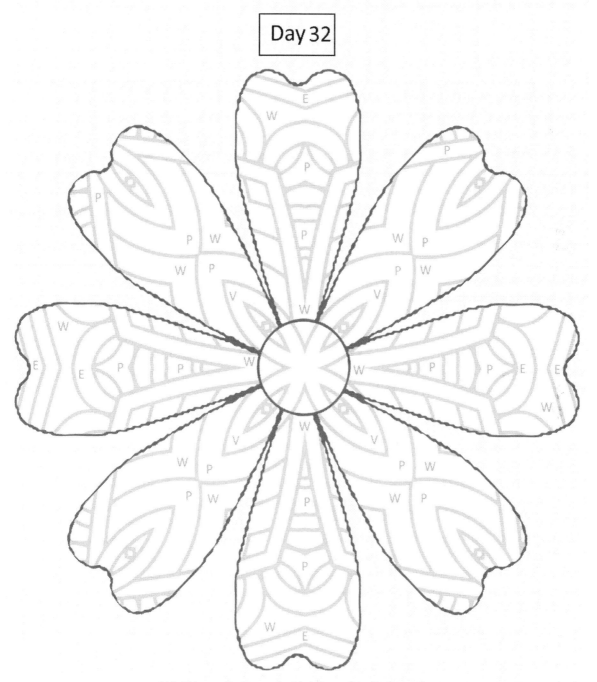

W=Water P=Protein V=Vitamins E=Exercise

THE BREAKTHROUGH JOURNAL

We cannot really think in one way and act in another... ~Thomas Troward

My #1 FOCUS for today is:

Date:

Breakfast	Calories	Protein	Carbs	Fat	Sugar
Time:					
Totals					

Lunch	Calories	Protein	Carbs	Fat	Sugar
Time:					
Totals					

Dinner	Calories	Protein	Carbs	Fat	Sugar
Time:					
Totals					

Snacks	Calories	Protein	Carbs	Fat	Sugar
Time:					
Time:					
Time:					
Totals					

Daily Totals					

Water (4 ounces per square)																
Protein (5 grams per square)																
Vitamins (1 vitamin per square)																
Exercise (10 minutes per square)																

Was my #1 FOCUS accomplished today? Y ☐ N ☐   My thoughts about today:

Decide and fill-in your #1 FOCUS on tomorrow's page.

THE BREAKTHROUGH JOURNAL

I am Decisive, Determined, Disciplined and Dynamic!

Day 33

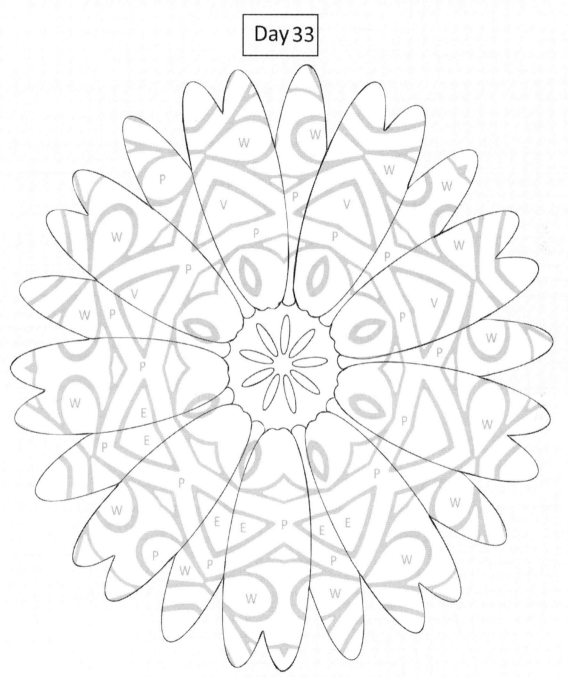

W=Water P=Protein V=Vitamins E=Exercise

THE BREAKTHROUGH JOURNAL

It doesn't matter where you are coming from. All that matters is where you are going. ~Brian Tracy

My #1 FOCUS for today is:

Date:

Breakfast	Calories	Protein	Carbs	Fat	Sugar
Time:					
Totals					

Lunch	Calories	Protein	Carbs	Fat	Sugar
Time:					
Totals					

Dinner	Calories	Protein	Carbs	Fat	Sugar
Time:					
Totals					

Snacks	Calories	Protein	Carbs	Fat	Sugar
Time:					
Time:					
Time:					
Totals					

Daily Totals					

Water (4 ounces per square)																	
Protein (5 grams per square)																	
Vitamins (1 vitamin per square)																	
Exercise (10 minutes per square)																	

Was my #1 FOCUS accomplished today? Y ☐ N ☐ **My thoughts about today:**

Decide and fill-in your #1 FOCUS on tomorrow's page.

I am Decisive, Determined, Disciplined and Dynamic!

Day 34

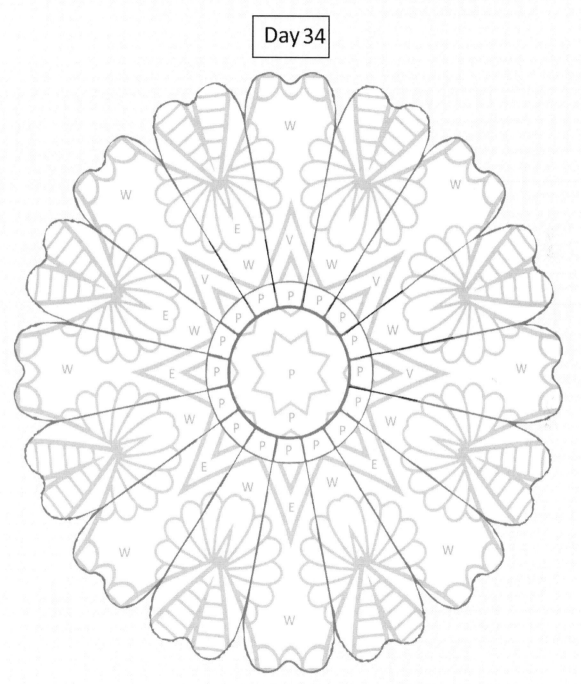

W=Water P=Protein V=Vitamins E=Exercise

THE BREAKTHROUGH JOURNAL

High achievement always takes place in the framework of high expectation. ~Charles Kettering

My #1 FOCUS for today is:

Date:

Breakfast	Calories	Protein	Carbs	Fat	Sugar
Time:					
Totals					

Lunch	Calories	Protein	Carbs	Fat	Sugar
Time:					
Totals					

Dinner	Calories	Protein	Carbs	Fat	Sugar
Time:					
Totals					

Snacks	Calories	Protein	Carbs	Fat	Sugar
Time:					
Time:					
Time:					
Totals					

Daily Totals					

Water (4 ounces per square)														
Protein (5 grams per square)														
Vitamins (1 vitamin per square)														
Exercise (10 minutes per square)														

Was my #1 FOCUS accomplished today? Y ☐ N ☐ My thoughts about today:

Decide and fill-in your #1 FOCUS on tomorrow's page.

I am Decisive, Determined, Disciplined and Dynamic!

Day 35

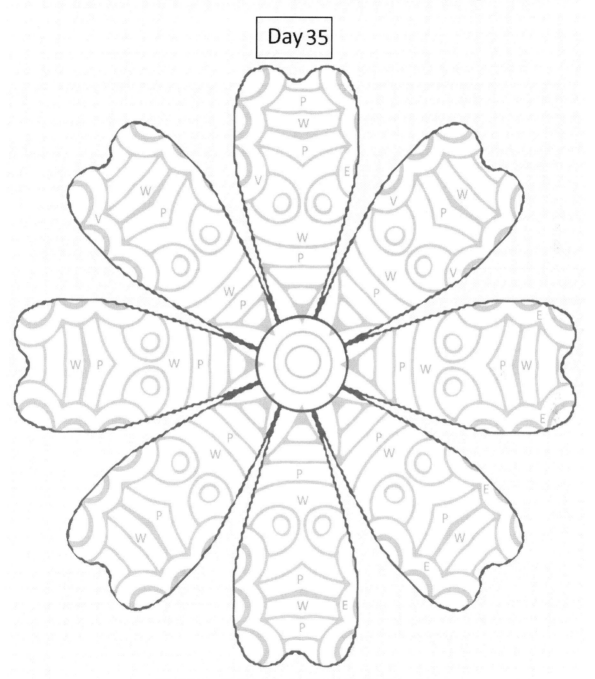

W=Water P=Protein V=Vitamins E=Exercise

WEEKLY REVIEW

Did I accomplish my goal this week?_____

What went well this week?_____

_____

_____

_____

What can be improved?_____

_____

_____

_____

My goal for the coming week is_____

_____

_____

My daily plan to accomplish this goal is_____

_____

_____

_____

_____

_____

_____

This is the behavior I will change this week_____

_____

THOUGHTS & IDEAS

THE BREAKTHROUGH JOURNAL

The path to success is to take massive, determined action. ~Tony Robbins

My #1 FOCUS for today is:

Date:

Breakfast	Calories	Protein	Carbs	Fat	Sugar
Time:					
Totals					

Lunch	Calories	Protein	Carbs	Fat	Sugar
Time:					
Totals					

Dinner	Calories	Protein	Carbs	Fat	Sugar
Time:					
Totals					

Snacks	Calories	Protein	Carbs	Fat	Sugar
Time:					
Time:					
Time:					
Totals					

Daily Totals					

Water (4 ounces per square)																
Protein (5 grams per square)																
Vitamins (1 vitamin per square)																
Exercise (10 minutes per square)																

Was my #1 FOCUS accomplished today? Y ☐ N ☐ **My thoughts about today:**

Decide and fill-in your #1 FOCUS on tomorrow's page.

THE BREAKTHROUGH JOURNAL

I am Decisive, Determined, Disciplined and Dynamic!

Day 36

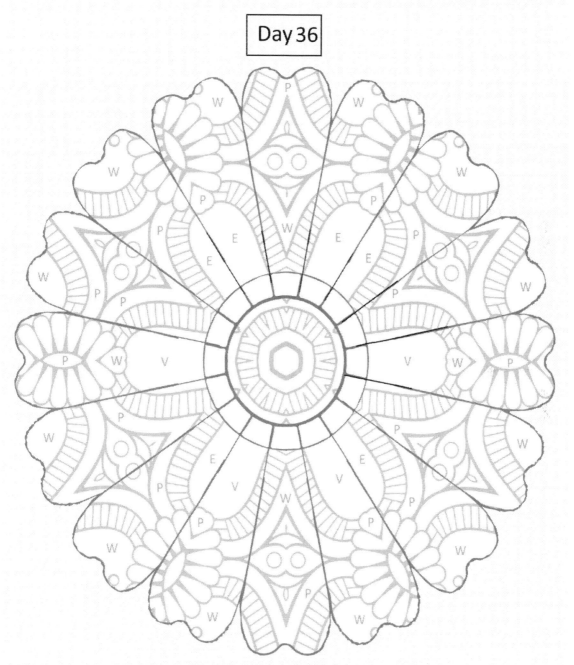

W=Water P=Protein V=Vitamins E=Exercise

THE BREAKTHROUGH JOURNAL

Whatever you dwell on in the conscious grows in your experience. ~Brian Tracy

My #1 FOCUS for today is:

Date:

Breakfast	Calories	Protein	Carbs	Fat	Sugar
Time:					
Totals					

Lunch	Calories	Protein	Carbs	Fat	Sugar
Time:					
Totals					

Dinner	Calories	Protein	Carbs	Fat	Sugar
Time:					
Totals					

Snacks	Calories	Protein	Carbs	Fat	Sugar
Time:					
Time:					
Time:					
Totals					

Daily Totals					

Water (4 ounces per square)																		
Protein (5 grams per square)																		
Vitamins (1 vitamin per square)																		
Exercise (10 minutes per square)																		

Was my #1 FOCUS accomplished today? Y ☐ N ☐ **My thoughts about today:**

Decide and fill-in your #1 FOCUS on tomorrow's page.

THE BREAKTHROUGH JOURNAL

I am Decisive, Determined, Disciplined and Dynamic!

Day 37

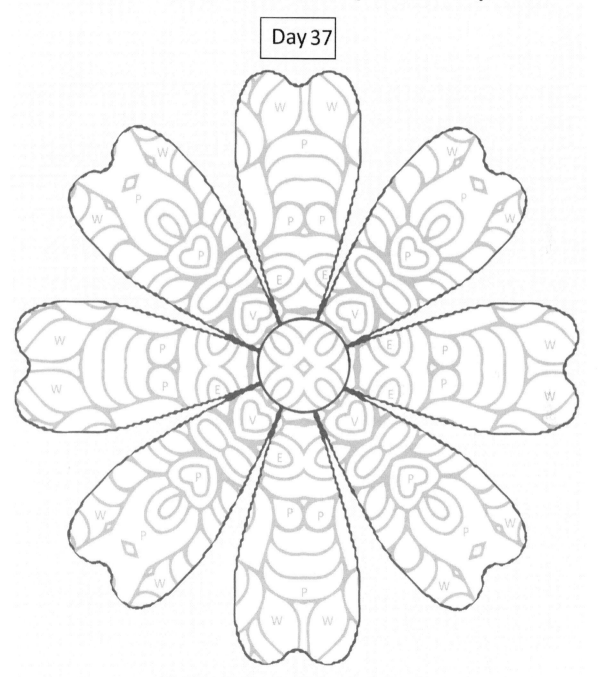

W=Water P=Protein V=Vitamins E=Exercise

THE BREAKTHROUGH JOURNAL

Happiness depends more on the inward disposition of mind than on outward circumstances. ~Benjamin Franklin

My #1 FOCUS for today is:

Date:

Breakfast	Calories	Protein	Carbs	Fat	Sugar
Time:					
Totals					

Lunch	Calories	Protein	Carbs	Fat	Sugar
Time:					
Totals					

Dinner	Calories	Protein	Carbs	Fat	Sugar
Time:					
Totals					

Snacks	Calories	Protein	Carbs	Fat	Sugar
Time:					
Time:					
Time:					
Totals					

Daily Totals					

Water (4 ounces per square)																		
Protein (5 grams per square)																		
Vitamins (1 vitamin per square)																		
Exercise (10 minutes per square)																		

Was my #1 FOCUS accomplished today? Y ☐ N ☐   My thoughts about today:

Decide and fill-in your #1 FOCUS on tomorrow's page.

THE BREAKTHROUGH JOURNAL

I am Decisive, Determined, Disciplined and Dynamic!

Day 38

W=Water P=Protein V=Vitamins E=Exercise

THE BREAKTHROUGH JOURNAL

You change your life by changing your heart. ~Max Lucado

My #1 FOCUS for today is:

Date:

Breakfast	Calories	Protein	Carbs	Fat	Sugar
Time:					
Totals					

Lunch	Calories	Protein	Carbs	Fat	Sugar
Time:					
Totals					

Dinner	Calories	Protein	Carbs	Fat	Sugar
Time:					
Totals					

Snacks	Calories	Protein	Carbs	Fat	Sugar
Time:					
Time:					
Time:					
Totals					

Daily Totals					

Water (4 ounces per square)																
Protein (5 grams per square)																
Vitamins (1 vitamin per square)																
Exercise (10 minutes per square)																

Was my #1 FOCUS accomplished today? Y ☐ N ☐   My thoughts about today:

Decide and fill-in your #1 FOCUS on tomorrow's page.

I am Decisive, Determined, Disciplined and Dynamic!

Day 39

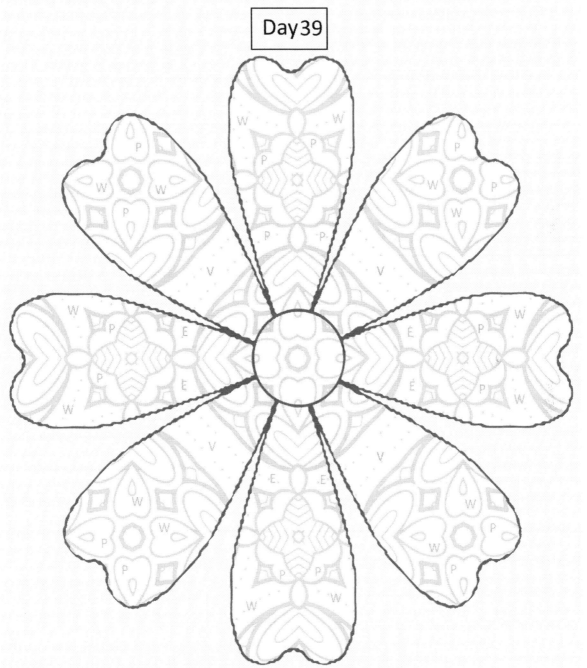

W=Water P=Protein V=Vitamins E=Exercise

THE BREAKTHROUGH JOURNAL

Effort only fully releases its reward after a person refuses to quit. ~Napoleon Hill

My #1 FOCUS for today is:

Date:

Breakfast	Calories	Protein	Carbs	Fat	Sugar
Time:					
Totals					

Lunch	Calories	Protein	Carbs	Fat	Sugar
Time:					
Totals					

Dinner	Calories	Protein	Carbs	Fat	Sugar
Time:					
Totals					

Snacks	Calories	Protein	Carbs	Fat	Sugar
Time:					
Time:					
Time:					
Totals					

Daily Totals					

Water (4 ounces per square)																
Protein (5 grams per square)																
Vitamins (1 vitamin per square)																
Exercise (10 minutes per square)																

Was my #1 FOCUS accomplished today? Y ☐ N ☐ **My thoughts about today:**

Decide and fill-in your #1 FOCUS on tomorrow's page.

I am Decisive, Determined, Disciplined and Dynamic!

Day 40

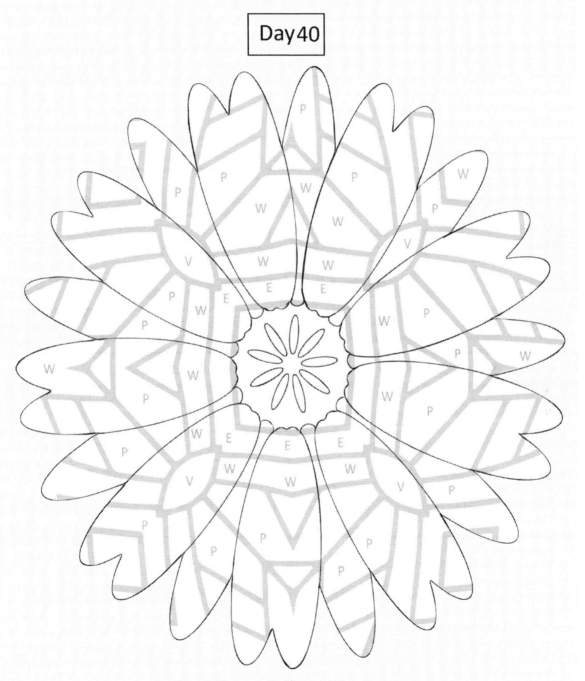

W=Water P=Protein V=Vitamins E=Exercise

THE BREAKTHROUGH JOURNAL

The man who views the world at 50 the same as he did at 20 has wasted 30 years of his life. ~Muhammad Ali

My #1 FOCUS for today is:

Date:

Breakfast	Calories	Protein	Carbs	Fat	Sugar
Time:					
Totals					

Lunch	Calories	Protein	Carbs	Fat	Sugar
Time:					
Totals					

Dinner	Calories	Protein	Carbs	Fat	Sugar
Time:					
Totals					

Snacks	Calories	Protein	Carbs	Fat	Sugar
Time:					
Time:					
Time:					
Totals					

Daily Totals					

Water (4 ounces per square)																		
Protein (5 grams per square)																		
Vitamins (1 vitamin per square)																		
Exercise (10 minutes per square)																		

Was my #1 FOCUS accomplished today? Y ☐ N ☐ **My thoughts about today:**

Decide and fill-in your #1 FOCUS on tomorrow's page.

I am Decisive, Determined, Disciplined and Dynamic!

Day 41

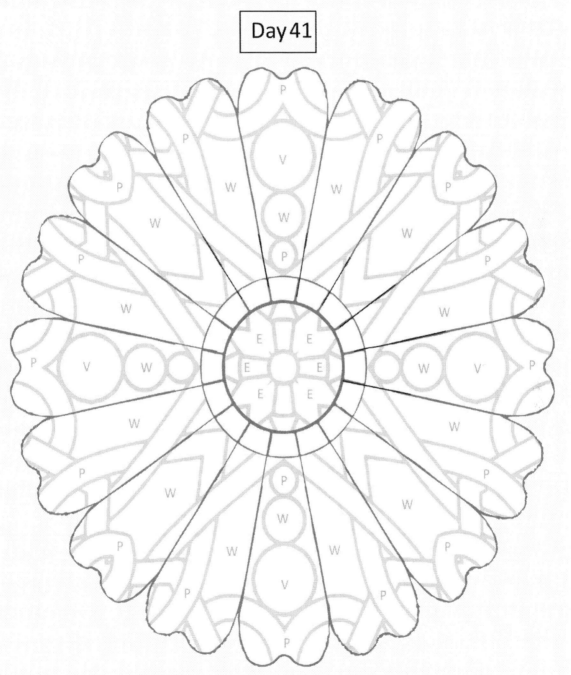

W=Water P=Protein V=Vitamins E=Exercise

THE BREAKTHROUGH JOURNAL

Action is the foundational key to all success. ~Pablo Picasso

My #1 FOCUS for today is:

Date:

Breakfast	Calories	Protein	Carbs	Fat	Sugar
Time:					
Totals					

Lunch	Calories	Protein	Carbs	Fat	Sugar
Time:					
Totals					

Dinner	Calories	Protein	Carbs	Fat	Sugar
Time:					
Totals					

Snacks	Calories	Protein	Carbs	Fat	Sugar
Time:					
Time:					
Time:					
Totals					

Daily Totals					

Water (4 ounces per square)															
Protein (5 grams per square)															
Vitamins (1 vitamin per square)															
Exercise (10 minutes per square)															

Was my #1 FOCUS accomplished today? Y ☐ N ☐ **My thoughts about today:**

Decide and fill-in your #1 FOCUS on tomorrow's page.

THE BREAKTHROUGH JOURNAL
I am Decisive, Determined, Disciplined and Dynamic!

Day 42

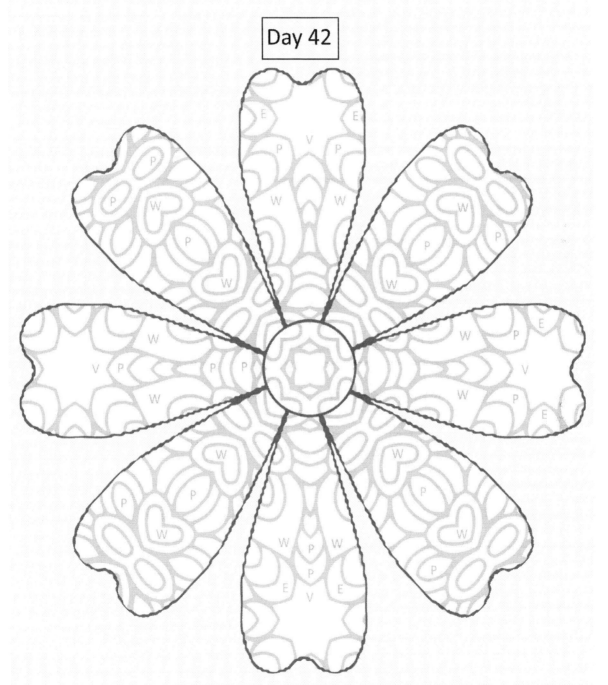

W=Water P=Protein V=Vitamins E=Exercise

WEEKLY REVIEW

Did I accomplish my goal this week?_____

What went well this week?_____
_____
_____
_____

What can be improved?_____
_____
_____
_____

My goal for the coming week is_____
_____
_____

My daily plan to accomplish this goal is_____
_____
_____
_____
_____
_____

This is the behavior I will change this week_____
_____

THOUGHTS & IDEAS

THE BREAKTHROUGH JOURNAL

Your success is your responsibility. Take the initiative, do the work, and persist to the end. ~Lorii Myers

My #1 FOCUS for today is:

Date:

Breakfast	Calories	Protein	Carbs	Fat	Sugar
Time:					
Totals					

Lunch	Calories	Protein	Carbs	Fat	Sugar
Time:					
Totals					

Dinner	Calories	Protein	Carbs	Fat	Sugar
Time:					
Totals					

Snacks	Calories	Protein	Carbs	Fat	Sugar
Time:					
Time:					
Time:					
Totals					

Daily Totals					

Water (4 ounces per square)																			
Protein (5 grams per square)																			
Vitamins (1 vitamin per square)																			
Exercise (10 minutes per square)																			

Was my #1 FOCUS accomplished today? Y ☐ N ☐ My thoughts about today:

Decide and fill-in your #1 FOCUS on tomorrow's page.

I am Decisive, Determined, Disciplined and Dynamic!

Day 43

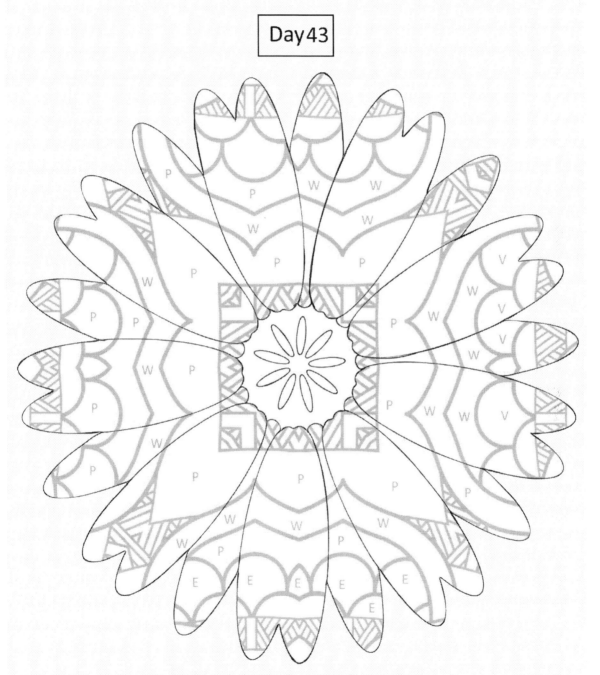

W=Water P=Protein V=Vitamins E=Exercise

THE BREAKTHROUGH JOURNAL

No idea, no matter how good, will work if it doesn't get used. ~Shad Helmstetter, Ph.D.

My #1 FOCUS for today is:

Date:

Breakfast	Calories	Protein	Carbs	Fat	Sugar
Time:					
Totals					

Lunch	Calories	Protein	Carbs	Fat	Sugar
Time:					
Totals					

Dinner	Calories	Protein	Carbs	Fat	Sugar
Time:					
Totals					

Snacks	Calories	Protein	Carbs	Fat	Sugar
Time:					
Time:					
Time:					
Totals					

Daily Totals					

Water (4 ounces per square)																				
Protein (5 grams per square)																				
Vitamins (1 vitamin per square)																				
Exercise (10 minutes per square)																				

Was my #1 FOCUS accomplished today? Y ☐ N ☐ **My thoughts about today:**

Decide and fill-in your #1 FOCUS on tomorrow's page.

I am Decisive, Determined, Disciplined and Dynamic!

Day 44

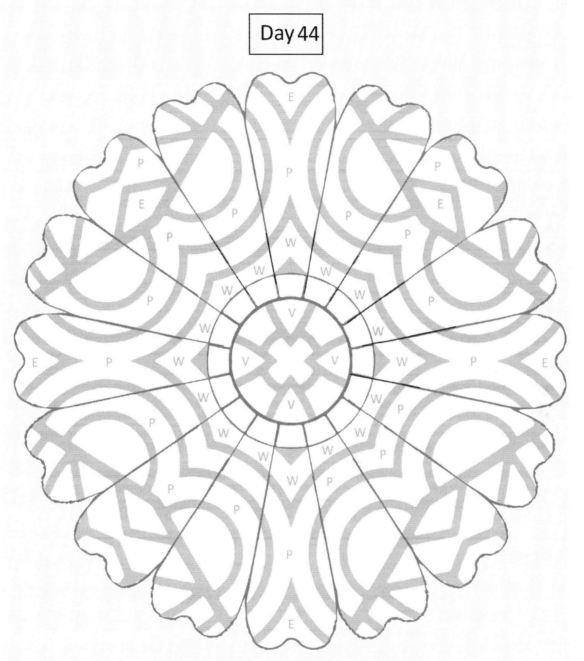

W=Water P=Protein V=Vitamins E=Exercise

THE BREAKTHROUGH JOURNAL

Make the most of yourself, for that is all there is of you. ~Ralph Waldo Emerson

My #1 FOCUS for today is:

Date:

Breakfast	Calories	Protein	Carbs	Fat	Sugar
Time:					
Totals					

Lunch	Calories	Protein	Carbs	Fat	Sugar
Time:					
Totals					

Dinner	Calories	Protein	Carbs	Fat	Sugar
Time:					
Totals					

Snacks	Calories	Protein	Carbs	Fat	Sugar
Time:					
Time:					
Time:					
Totals					

Daily Totals					

Water (4 ounces per square)		
Protein (5 grams per square)		
Vitamins (1 vitamin per square)		
Exercise (10 minutes per square)		

Was my #1 FOCUS accomplished today? Y ☐ N ☐ My thoughts about today:

Decide and fill-in your #1 FOCUS on tomorrow's page.

I am Decisive, Determined, Disciplined and Dynamic!

Day 45

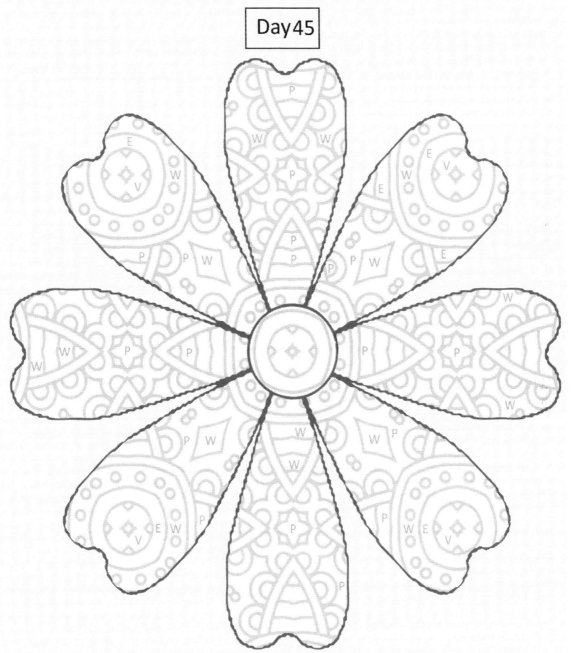

W=Water P=Protein V=Vitamins E=Exercise

THE BREAKTHROUGH JOURNAL

Argue for your limitations and, sure enough, they're yours. ~Richard Bach

My #1 FOCUS for today is:

Date:

Breakfast	Calories	Protein	Carbs	Fat	Sugar
Time:					
Totals					

Lunch	Calories	Protein	Carbs	Fat	Sugar
Time:					
Totals					

Dinner	Calories	Protein	Carbs	Fat	Sugar
Time:					
Totals					

Snacks	Calories	Protein	Carbs	Fat	Sugar
Time:					
Time:					
Time:					
Totals					

Daily Totals					

Water (4 ounces per square)																
Protein (5 grams per square)																
Vitamins (1 vitamin per square)																
Exercise (10 minutes per square)																

Was my #1 FOCUS accomplished today? Y ☐ N ☐ My thoughts about today:

Decide and fill-in your #1 FOCUS on tomorrow's page.

I am Decisive, Determined, Disciplined and Dynamic!

Day 46

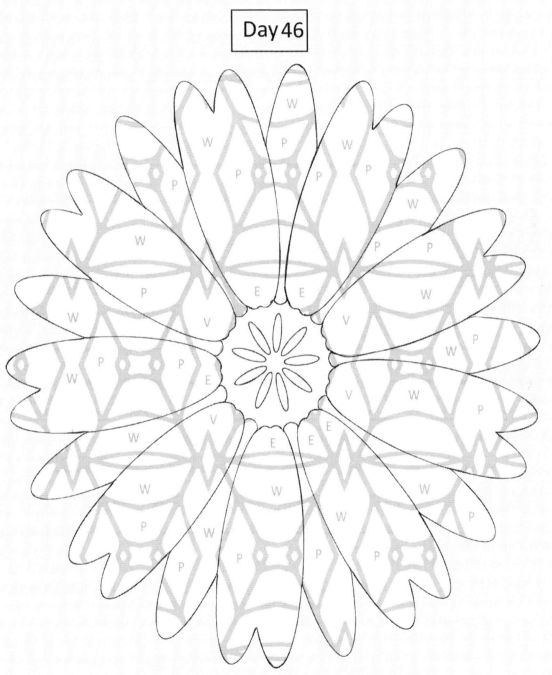

W=Water P=Protein V=Vitamins E=Exercise

THE BREAKTHROUGH JOURNAL

Whatever we expect with confidence becomes our own self-fulfilling prophecy. ~Brian Tracy

My #1 FOCUS for today is:

Date:

Breakfast	Calories	Protein	Carbs	Fat	Sugar
Time:					
Totals					

Lunch	Calories	Protein	Carbs	Fat	Sugar
Time:					
Totals					

Dinner	Calories	Protein	Carbs	Fat	Sugar
Time:					
Totals					

Snacks	Calories	Protein	Carbs	Fat	Sugar
Time:					
Time:					
Time:					
Totals					

Daily Totals					

Water (4 ounces per square)															
Protein (5 grams per square)															
Vitamins (1 vitamin per square)															
Exercise (10 minutes per square)															

Was my #1 FOCUS accomplished today? Y ☐ N ☐ **My thoughts about today:**

Decide and fill-in your #1 FOCUS on tomorrow's page.

THE BREAKTHROUGH JOURNAL
I am Decisive, Determined, Disciplined and Dynamic!

Day 47

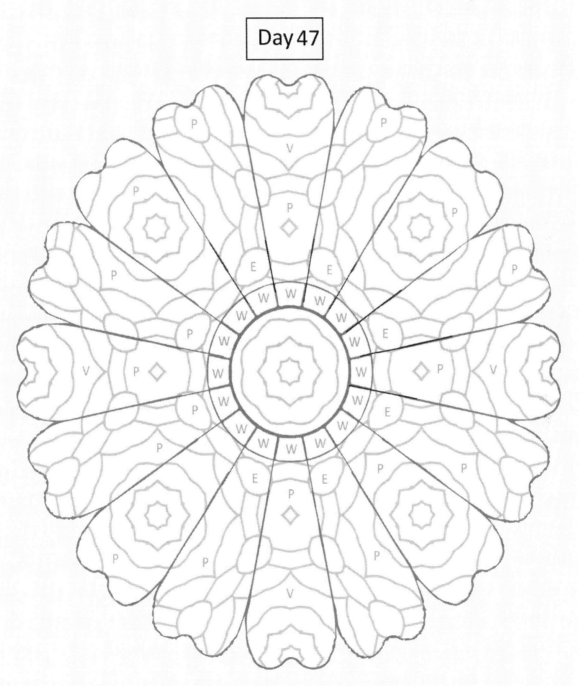

W=Water P=Protein V=Vitamins E=Exercise

THE BREAKTHROUGH JOURNAL

The trick is to enjoy life. Don't wish away your days, waiting for better ones ahead. ~Marjorie Pay Hinckley

My #1 FOCUS for today is:

Date:

Breakfast	Calories	Protein	Carbs	Fat	Sugar
Time:					
Totals					

Lunch	Calories	Protein	Carbs	Fat	Sugar
Time:					
Totals					

Dinner	Calories	Protein	Carbs	Fat	Sugar
Time:					
Totals					

Snacks	Calories	Protein	Carbs	Fat	Sugar
Time:					
Time:					
Time:					
Totals					

Daily Totals					

Water (4 ounces per square)																
Protein (5 grams per square)																
Vitamins (1 vitamin per square)																
Exercise (10 minutes per square)																

Was my #1 FOCUS accomplished today? Y ☐ N ☐ My thoughts about today:

Decide and fill-in your #1 FOCUS on tomorrow's page.

I am Decisive, Determined, Disciplined and Dynamic!

Day 48

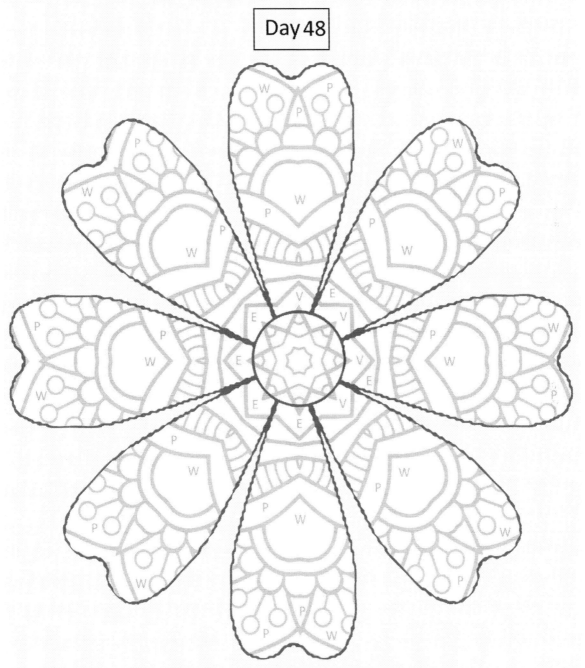

W=Water P=Protein V=Vitamins E=Exercise

THE BREAKTHROUGH JOURNAL

Willpower is the unflinching purpose to see a task through to completion. ~Jerry Bruckner

My #1 FOCUS for today is:

Date:

Breakfast	Calories	Protein	Carbs	Fat	Sugar
Time:					
Totals					

Lunch	Calories	Protein	Carbs	Fat	Sugar
Time:					
Totals					

Dinner	Calories	Protein	Carbs	Fat	Sugar
Time:					
Totals					

Snacks	Calories	Protein	Carbs	Fat	Sugar
Time:					
Time:					
Time:					
Totals					

Daily Totals					

Water (4 ounces per square)	
Protein (5 grams per square)	
Vitamins (1 vitamin per square)	
Exercise (10 minutes per square)	

Was my #1 FOCUS accomplished today? Y ☐ N ☐ **My thoughts about today:**

Decide and fill-in your #1 FOCUS on tomorrow's page.

I am Decisive, Determined, Disciplined and Dynamic!

Day 49

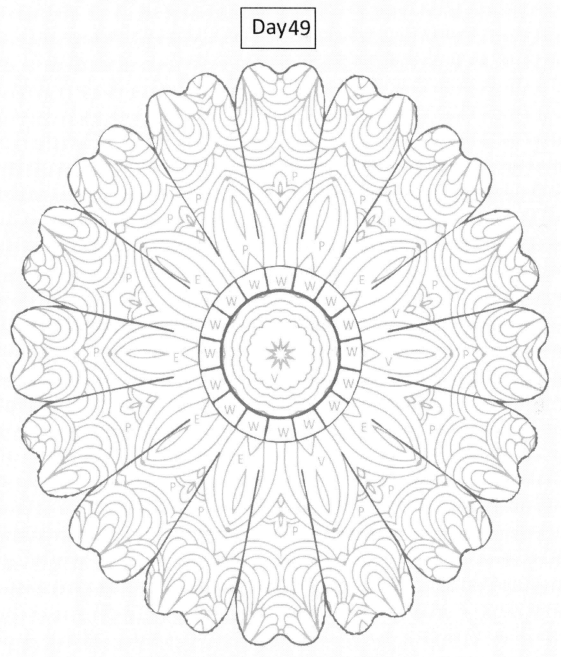

W=Water P=Protein V=Vitamins E=Exercise

WEEKLY REVIEW

Did I accomplish my goal this week?_____

What went well this week?_____

_____

_____

_____

What can be improved?_____

_____

_____

_____

My goal for the coming week is_____

_____

_____

My daily plan to accomplish this goal is_____

_____

_____

_____

_____

_____

This is the behavior I will change this week_____

_____

THOUGHTS & IDEAS

THE BREAKTHROUGH JOURNAL

To improve our conditions we must first improve ourselves. ~Charles F. Haanel

My #1 FOCUS for today is:

Date:

Breakfast	Calories	Protein	Carbs	Fat	Sugar
Time:					
Totals					

Lunch	Calories	Protein	Carbs	Fat	Sugar
Time:					
Totals					

Dinner	Calories	Protein	Carbs	Fat	Sugar
Time:					
Totals					

Snacks	Calories	Protein	Carbs	Fat	Sugar
Time:					
Time:					
Time:					
Totals					

Daily Totals					

Water (4 ounces per square)															
Protein (5 grams per square)															
Vitamins (1 vitamin per square)															
Exercise (10 minutes per square)															

Was my #1 FOCUS accomplished today? Y ☐ N ☐ **My thoughts about today:**

Decide and fill-in your #1 FOCUS on tomorrow's page.

I am Decisive, Determined, Disciplined and Dynamic!

Day 50

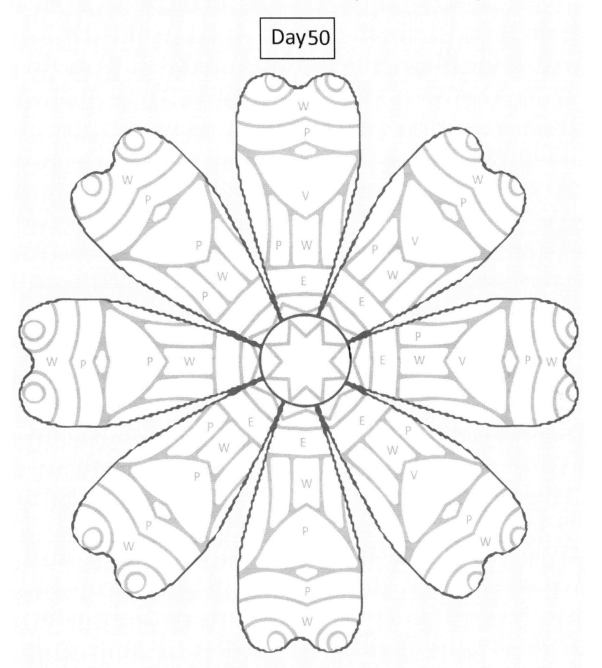

W=Water P=Protein V=Vitamins E=Exercise

THE BREAKTHROUGH JOURNAL

We are only failures in life when we give up and stop trying. If you fail, get up and try again. ~Lailah Gifty Akita

My #1 FOCUS for today is:

Date:

Breakfast	Calories	Protein	Carbs	Fat	Sugar
Time:					
Totals					

Lunch	Calories	Protein	Carbs	Fat	Sugar
Time:					
Totals					

Dinner	Calories	Protein	Carbs	Fat	Sugar
Time:					
Totals					

Snacks	Calories	Protein	Carbs	Fat	Sugar
Time:					
Time:					
Time:					
Totals					

Daily Totals					

Water (4 ounces per square)																
Protein (5 grams per square)																
Vitamins (1 vitamin per square)																
Exercise (10 minutes per square)																

Was my #1 FOCUS accomplished today? Y ☐ N ☐   **My thoughts about today:**

Decide and fill-in your #1 FOCUS on tomorrow's page.

I am Decisive, Determined, Disciplined and Dynamic!

Day 51

W=Water P=Protein V=Vitamins E=Exercise

THE BREAKTHROUGH JOURNAL

Belief in limitation is the one and only thing that causes limitation. ~Thomas Troward

My #1 FOCUS for today is:

Date:

Breakfast	Calories	Protein	Carbs	Fat	Sugar
Time:					
Totals					

Lunch	Calories	Protein	Carbs	Fat	Sugar
Time:					
Totals					

Dinner	Calories	Protein	Carbs	Fat	Sugar
Time:					
Totals					

Snacks	Calories	Protein	Carbs	Fat	Sugar
Time:					
Time:					
Time:					
Totals					

Daily Totals					

Water (4 ounces per square)	
Protein (5 grams per square)	
Vitamins (1 vitamin per square)	
Exercise (10 minutes per square)	

Was my #1 FOCUS accomplished today? Y ☐ N ☐ My thoughts about today:

Decide and fill-in your #1 FOCUS on tomorrow's page.

THE BREAKTHROUGH JOURNAL

I am Decisive, Determined, Disciplined and Dynamic!

Day 52

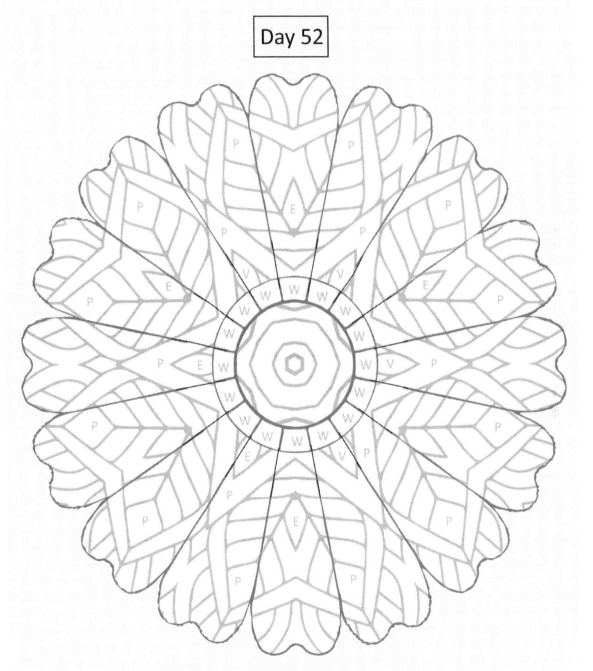

W=Water P=Protein V=Vitamins E=Exercise

THE BREAKTHROUGH JOURNAL

Persistence breaks down resistance. ~Jerry Bruckner

My #1 FOCUS for today is:

Date:

Breakfast	Calories	Protein	Carbs	Fat	Sugar
Time:					
Totals					

Lunch	Calories	Protein	Carbs	Fat	Sugar
Time:					
Totals					

Dinner	Calories	Protein	Carbs	Fat	Sugar
Time:					
Totals					

Snacks	Calories	Protein	Carbs	Fat	Sugar
Time:					
Time:					
Time:					
Totals					

Daily Totals					

Water (4 ounces per square)																
Protein (5 grams per square)																
Vitamins (1 vitamin per square)																
Exercise (10 minutes per square)																

Was my #1 FOCUS accomplished today? Y ☐ N ☐ **My thoughts about today:**

Decide and fill-in your #1 FOCUS on tomorrow's page.

I am Decisive, Determined, Disciplined and Dynamic!

Day 53

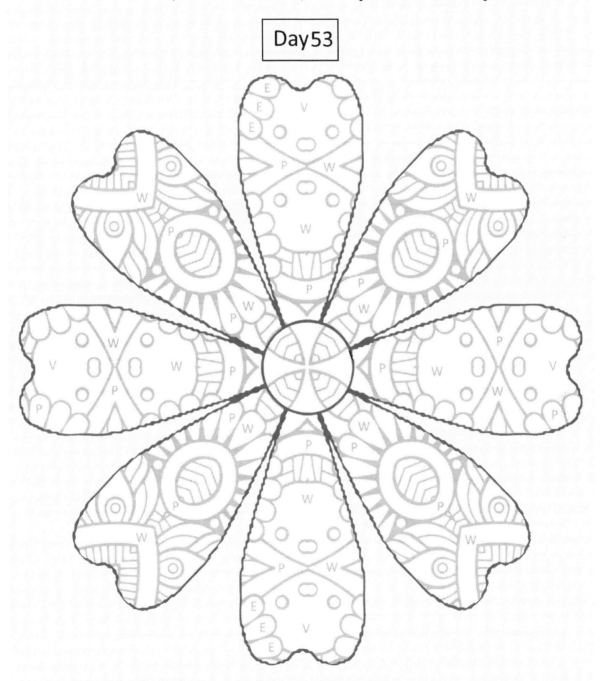

W=Water P=Protein V=Vitamins E=Exercise

THE BREAKTHROUGH JOURNAL

Life is a mirror and will reflect back to the thinker what he thinks into it. ~Ernest Holmes

My #1 FOCUS for today is:

Date:

Breakfast	Calories	Protein	Carbs	Fat	Sugar
Time:					
Totals					

Lunch	Calories	Protein	Carbs	Fat	Sugar
Time:					
Totals					

Dinner	Calories	Protein	Carbs	Fat	Sugar
Time:					
Totals					

Snacks	Calories	Protein	Carbs	Fat	Sugar
Time:					
Time:					
Time:					
Totals					

Daily Totals					

Water (4 ounces per square)																	
Protein (5 grams per square)																	
Vitamins (1 vitamin per square)																	
Exercise (10 minutes per square)																	

Was my #1 FOCUS accomplished today? Y ☐ N ☐ **My thoughts about today:**

Decide and fill-in your #1 FOCUS on tomorrow's page.

I am Decisive, Determined, Disciplined and Dynamic!

Day 54

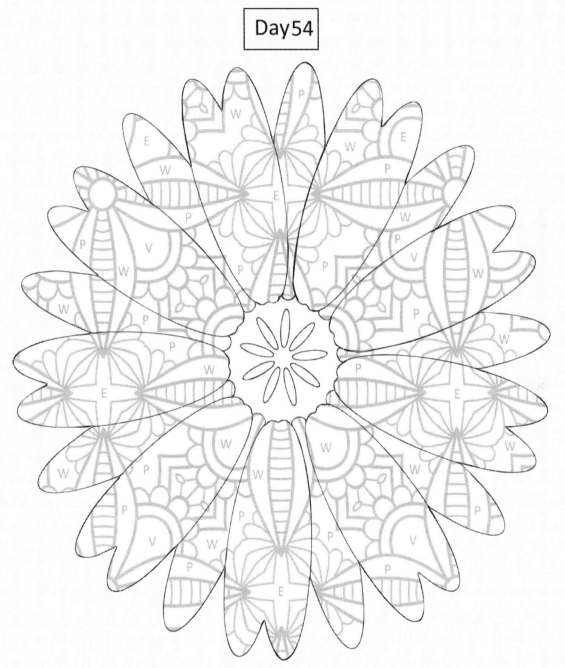

W=Water P=Protein V=Vitamins E=Exercise

THE BREAKTHROUGH JOURNAL

When someone criticizes you, it defines who they are, not who you are. ~Marie Forleo

My #1 FOCUS for today is:

Date:

Breakfast	Calories	Protein	Carbs	Fat	Sugar
Time:					
Totals					

Lunch	Calories	Protein	Carbs	Fat	Sugar
Time:					
Totals					

Dinner	Calories	Protein	Carbs	Fat	Sugar
Time:					
Totals					

Snacks	Calories	Protein	Carbs	Fat	Sugar
Time:					
Time:					
Time:					
Totals					

Daily Totals					

Water (4 ounces per square)																
Protein (5 grams per square)																
Vitamins (1 vitamin per square)																
Exercise (10 minutes per square)																

Was my #1 FOCUS accomplished today? Y ☐ N ☐ **My thoughts about today:**

Decide and fill-in your #1 FOCUS on tomorrow's page.

I am Decisive, Determined, Disciplined and Dynamic!

Day 55

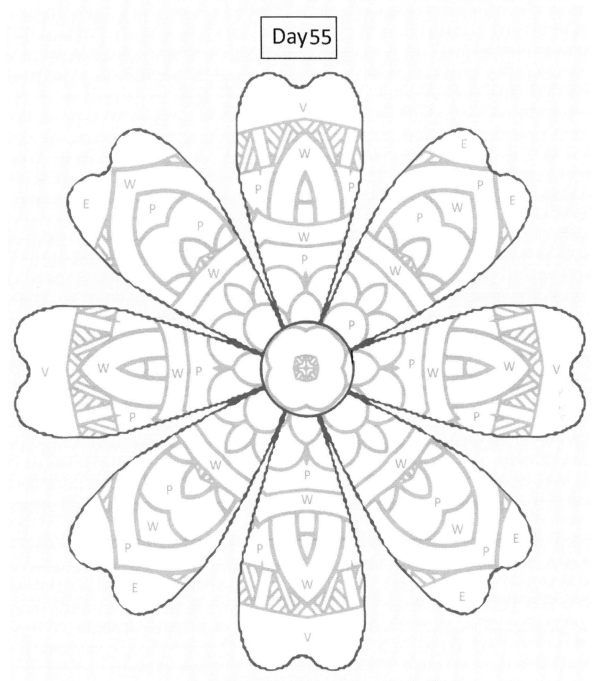

W=Water P=Protein V=Vitamins E=Exercise

THE BREAKTHROUGH JOURNAL

Strength doesn't come from what you can do. It comes from overcoming the things you once thought you couldn't. ~Rikki Rogers

My #1 FOCUS for today is:

Date:

Breakfast	Calories	Protein	Carbs	Fat	Sugar
Time:					
Totals					

Lunch	Calories	Protein	Carbs	Fat	Sugar
Time:					
Totals					

Dinner	Calories	Protein	Carbs	Fat	Sugar
Time:					
Totals					

Snacks	Calories	Protein	Carbs	Fat	Sugar
Time:					
Time:					
Time:					
Totals					

Daily Totals					

Water (4 ounces per square)																				
Protein (5 grams per square)																				
Vitamins (1 vitamin per square)																				
Exercise (10 minutes per square)																				

Was my #1 FOCUS accomplished today? Y ☐ N ☐ **My thoughts about today:**

Decide and fill-in your #1 FOCUS on tomorrow's page.

THE BREAKTHROUGH JOURNAL

I am Decisive, Determined, Disciplined and Dynamic!

Day 56

W=Water P=Protein V=Vitamins E=Exercise

WEEKLY REVIEW

Did I accomplish my goal this week?_____

What went well this week?_____
_____
_____
_____

What can be improved?_____
_____
_____
_____

My goal for the coming week is_____
_____
_____

My daily plan to accomplish this goal is_____
_____
_____
_____
_____
_____

This is the behavior I will change this week_____
_____

MONTHLY REVIEW

Date:_____

Weight:_____

Bust Measurement:_____

Waist Measurement:_____

Hips Measurement:_____

My major accomplishments during the last 4 weeks were_____

_____

_____

_____

What do I need to improve during the next 4 weeks?_____

_____

_____

My goal for the next 4 weeks is_____

_____

_____

My weekly plan to accomplish this goal during the next 4 weeks is_____

_____

_____

_____

_____

THE BREAKTHROUGH JOURNAL

Self-affirm—build yourself up with honest and genuine praise. ~Lorii Myers

My #1 FOCUS for today is:

Date:

Breakfast	Calories	Protein	Carbs	Fat	Sugar
Time:					
Totals					

Lunch	Calories	Protein	Carbs	Fat	Sugar
Time:					
Totals					

Dinner	Calories	Protein	Carbs	Fat	Sugar
Time:					
Totals					

Snacks	Calories	Protein	Carbs	Fat	Sugar
Time:					
Time:					
Time:					
Totals					

Daily Totals					

Water (4 ounces per square)																
Protein (5 grams per square)																
Vitamins (1 vitamin per square)																
Exercise (10 minutes per square)																

Was my #1 FOCUS accomplished today? Y ☐ N ☐ **My thoughts about today:**

Decide and fill-in your #1 FOCUS on tomorrow's page.

THE BREAKTHROUGH JOURNAL

I am Decisive, Determined, Disciplined and Dynamic!

Day 57

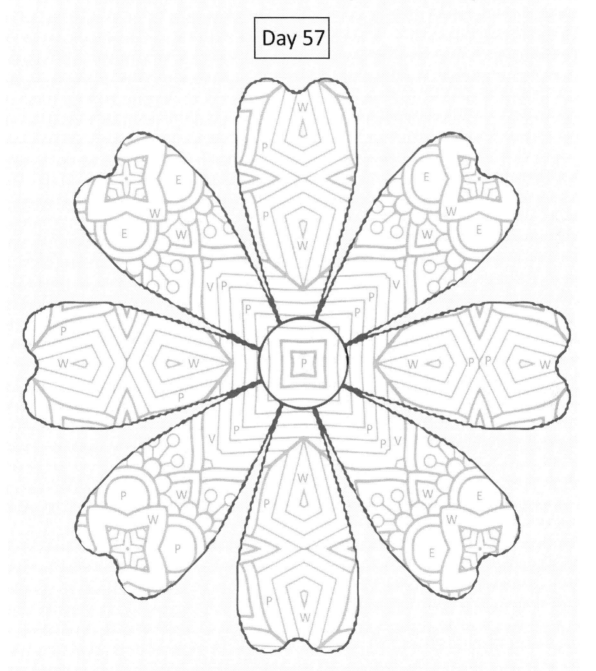

W=Water P=Protein V=Vitamins E=Exercise

THE BREAKTHROUGH JOURNAL

Problems cannot be solved by the same level of thinking that created them. ~Albert Einstein

My #1 FOCUS for today is:

Date:

Breakfast	Calories	Protein	Carbs	Fat	Sugar
Time:					
Totals					

Lunch	Calories	Protein	Carbs	Fat	Sugar
Time:					
Totals					

Dinner	Calories	Protein	Carbs	Fat	Sugar
Time:					
Totals					

Snacks	Calories	Protein	Carbs	Fat	Sugar
Time:					
Time:					
Time:					
Totals					

Daily Totals					

Water (4 ounces per square)																				
Protein (5 grams per square)																				
Vitamins (1 vitamin per square)																				
Exercise (10 minutes per square)																				

Was my #1 FOCUS accomplished today? Y ☐ N ☐   My thoughts about today:

Decide and fill-in your #1 FOCUS on tomorrow's page.

THE BREAKTHROUGH JOURNAL

I am Decisive, Determined, Disciplined and Dynamic!

Day 58

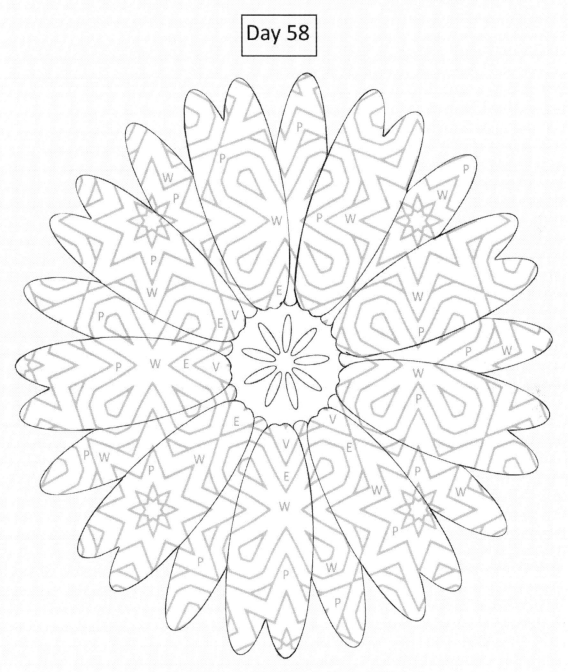

W=Water P=Protein V=Vitamins E=Exercise

THE BREAKTHROUGH JOURNAL

Most people are about as happy as they make up their minds to be. ~Abraham Lincoln

My #1 FOCUS for today is:

Date:

Breakfast	Calories	Protein	Carbs	Fat	Sugar
Time:					
Totals					

Lunch	Calories	Protein	Carbs	Fat	Sugar
Time:					
Totals					

Dinner	Calories	Protein	Carbs	Fat	Sugar
Time:					
Totals					

Snacks	Calories	Protein	Carbs	Fat	Sugar
Time:					
Time:					
Time:					
Totals					

Daily Totals					

Water (4 ounces per square)	
Protein (5 grams per square)	
Vitamins (1 vitamin per square)	
Exercise (10 minutes per square)	

Was my #1 FOCUS accomplished today? Y ☐ N ☐ My thoughts about today:

Decide and fill-in your #1 FOCUS on tomorrow's page.

I am Decisive, Determined, Disciplined and Dynamic!

Day 59

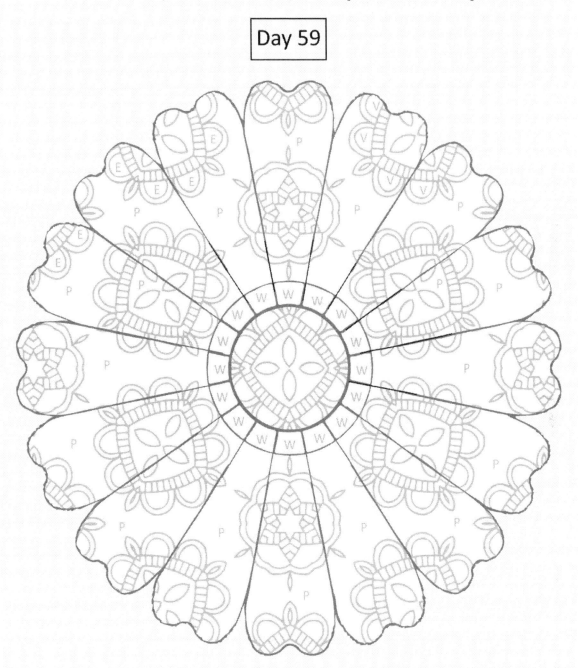

W=Water P=Protein V=Vitamins E=Exercise

THE BREAKTHROUGH JOURNAL

How am I going to live today in order to create the tomorrow I'm committed to? ~Tony Robbins

My #1 FOCUS for today is:

Date:

Breakfast	Calories	Protein	Carbs	Fat	Sugar
Time:					
Totals					

Lunch	Calories	Protein	Carbs	Fat	Sugar
Time:					
Totals					

Dinner	Calories	Protein	Carbs	Fat	Sugar
Time:					
Totals					

Snacks	Calories	Protein	Carbs	Fat	Sugar
Time:					
Time:					
Time:					
Totals					

Daily Totals					

Water (4 ounces per square)																		
Protein (5 grams per square)																		
Vitamins (1 vitamin per square)																		
Exercise (10 minutes per square)																		

Was my #1 FOCUS accomplished today? Y ☐ N ☐ My thoughts about today:

Decide and fill-in your #1 FOCUS on tomorrow's page.

THE BREAKTHROUGH JOURNAL

I am Decisive, Determined, Disciplined and Dynamic!

Day 60

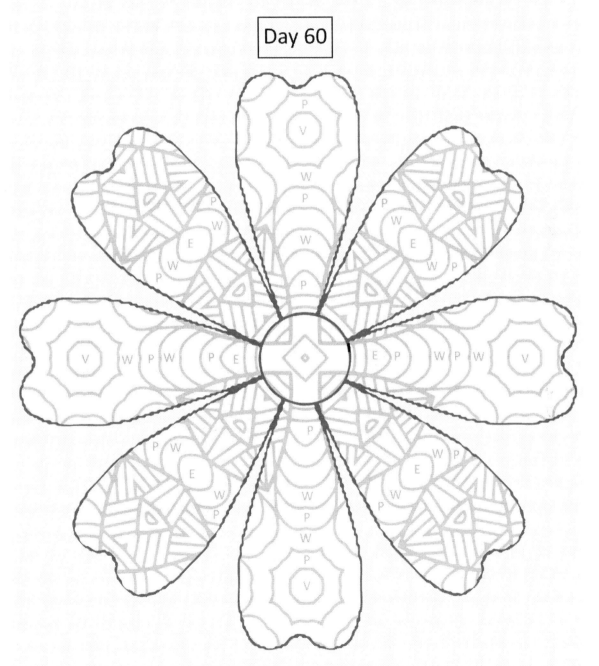

W=Water P=Protein V=Vitamins E=Exercise

THE BREAKTHROUGH JOURNAL

Life is 10% of what happens to me and 90% of how I react to it. ~John Maxwell

My #1 FOCUS for today is:

Date:

Breakfast	Calories	Protein	Carbs	Fat	Sugar
Time:					
Totals					

Lunch	Calories	Protein	Carbs	Fat	Sugar
Time:					
Totals					

Dinner	Calories	Protein	Carbs	Fat	Sugar
Time:					
Totals					

Snacks	Calories	Protein	Carbs	Fat	Sugar
Time:					
Time:					
Time:					
Totals					

Daily Totals					

Water (4 ounces per square)																
Protein (5 grams per square)																
Vitamins (1 vitamin per square)																
Exercise (10 minutes per square)																

Was my #1 FOCUS accomplished today? Y ☐ N ☐ My thoughts about today:

Decide and fill-in your #1 FOCUS on tomorrow's page.

THE BREAKTHROUGH JOURNAL

I am Decisive, Determined, Disciplined and Dynamic!

Day 61

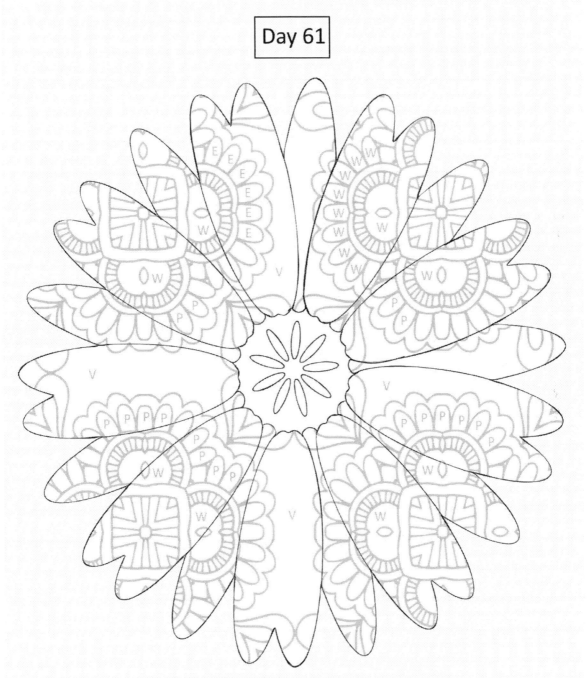

W=Water P=Protein V=Vitamins E=Exercise

THE BREAKTHROUGH JOURNAL

Many of life's failures are people who did not realize how close they were to success when they gave up. ~Thomas A. Edison

My #1 FOCUS for today is:

Date:

Breakfast	Calories	Protein	Carbs	Fat	Sugar
Time:					
Totals					

Lunch	Calories	Protein	Carbs	Fat	Sugar
Time:					
Totals					

Dinner	Calories	Protein	Carbs	Fat	Sugar
Time:					
Totals					

Snacks	Calories	Protein	Carbs	Fat	Sugar
Time:					
Time:					
Time:					
Totals					

Daily Totals					

Water (4 ounces per square)															
Protein (5 grams per square)															
Vitamins (1 vitamin per square)															
Exercise (10 minutes per square)															

Was my #1 FOCUS accomplished today? Y ☐ N ☐ **My thoughts about today:**

Decide and fill-in your #1 FOCUS on tomorrow's page.

THE BREAKTHROUGH JOURNAL
I am Decisive, Determined, Disciplined and Dynamic!

Day 62

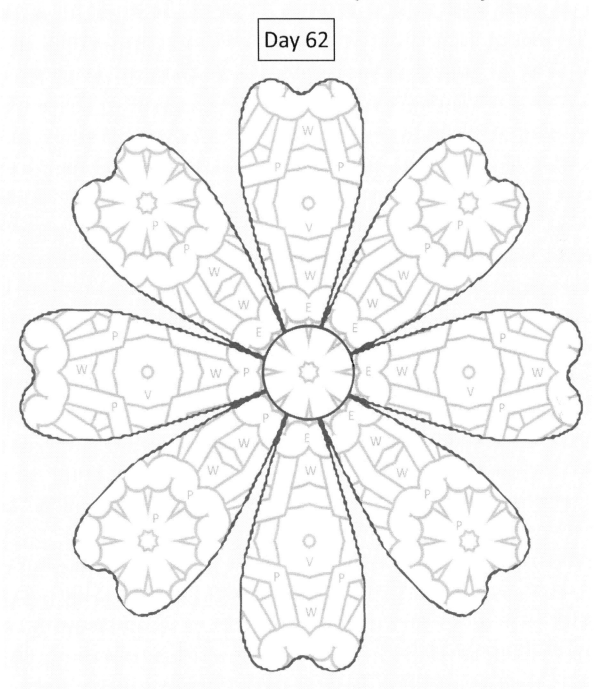

W=Water P=Protein V=Vitamins E=Exercise

THE BREAKTHROUGH JOURNAL

They can because they think they can. ~Virgil

My #1 FOCUS for today is:

Date:

Breakfast	Calories	Protein	Carbs	Fat	Sugar
Time:					
Totals					

Lunch	Calories	Protein	Carbs	Fat	Sugar
Time:					
Totals					

Dinner	Calories	Protein	Carbs	Fat	Sugar
Time:					
Totals					

Snacks	Calories	Protein	Carbs	Fat	Sugar
Time:					
Time:					
Time:					
Totals					

Daily Totals					

Water (4 ounces per square)																				
Protein (5 grams per square)																				
Vitamins (1 vitamin per square)																				
Exercise (10 minutes per square)																				

Was my #1 FOCUS accomplished today? Y ☐ N ☐ **My thoughts about today:**

Decide and fill-in your #1 FOCUS on tomorrow's page.

I am Decisive, Determined, Disciplined and Dynamic!

Day 63

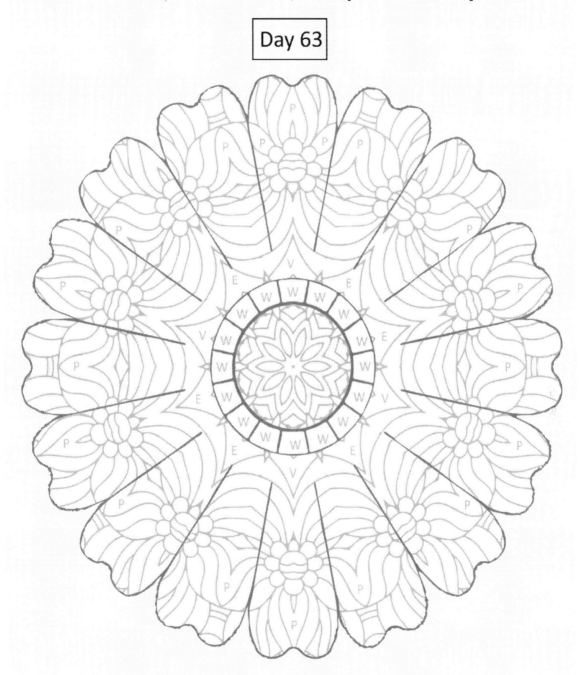

W=Water P=Protein V=Vitamins E=Exercise

WEEKLY REVIEW

Did I accomplish my goal this week?_____

What went well this week?_____

_____

_____

_____

What can be improved?_____

_____

_____

_____

My goal for the coming week is_____

_____

_____

My daily plan to accomplish this goal is_____

_____

_____

_____

_____

_____

This is the behavior I will change this week_____

_____

THOUGHTS & IDEAS

THE BREAKTHROUGH JOURNAL

He who has a why to live can bear almost any how. ~Friedrich Nietzsche

My #1 FOCUS for today is:

Date:

Breakfast	Calories	Protein	Carbs	Fat	Sugar
Time:					
Totals					

Lunch	Calories	Protein	Carbs	Fat	Sugar
Time:					
Totals					

Dinner	Calories	Protein	Carbs	Fat	Sugar
Time:					
Totals					

Snacks	Calories	Protein	Carbs	Fat	Sugar
Time:					
Time:					
Time:					
Totals					

Daily Totals					

Water (4 ounces per square)																			
Protein (5 grams per square)																			
Vitamins (1 vitamin per square)																			
Exercise (10 minutes per square)																			

Was my #1 FOCUS accomplished today? Y ☐ N ☐ **My thoughts about today:**

Decide and fill-in your #1 FOCUS on tomorrow's page.

THE BREAKTHROUGH JOURNAL

I am Decisive, Determined, Disciplined and Dynamic!

Day 64

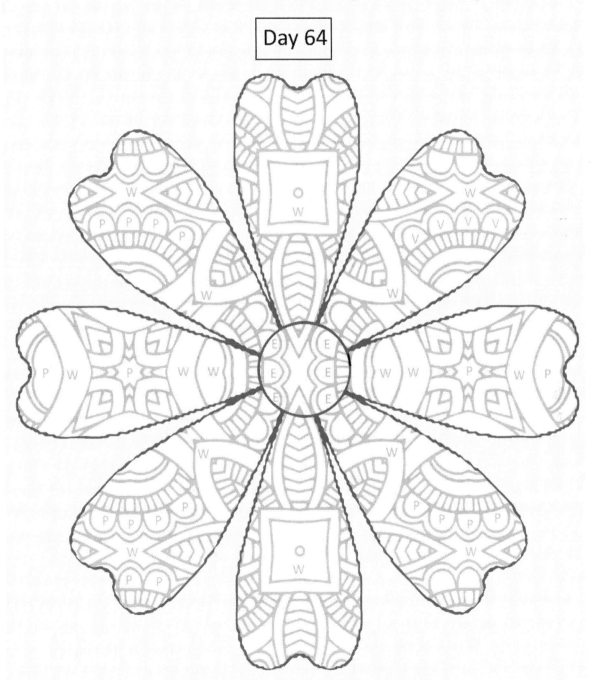

W=Water P=Protein V=Vitamins E=Exercise

THE BREAKTHROUGH JOURNAL

If what you are doing is not moving you towards your goals, then it's moving you away from your goals. ~Brian Tracy

My #1 FOCUS for today is:

Date:

Breakfast	Calories	Protein	Carbs	Fat	Sugar
Time:					
Totals					

Lunch	Calories	Protein	Carbs	Fat	Sugar
Time:					
Totals					

Dinner	Calories	Protein	Carbs	Fat	Sugar
Time:					
Totals					

Snacks	Calories	Protein	Carbs	Fat	Sugar
Time:					
Time:					
Time:					
Totals					

Daily Totals					

Water (4 ounces per square)																				
Protein (5 grams per square)																				
Vitamins (1 vitamin per square)																				
Exercise (10 minutes per square)																				

Was my #1 FOCUS accomplished today? Y ☐ N ☐ My thoughts about today:

Decide and fill-in your #1 FOCUS on tomorrow's page.

I am Decisive, Determined, Disciplined and Dynamic!

Day 65

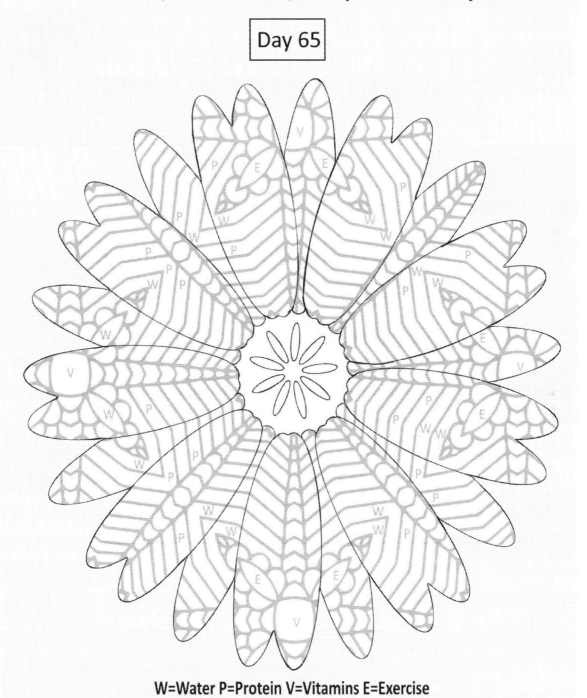

W=Water P=Protein V=Vitamins E=Exercise

THE BREAKTHROUGH JOURNAL

Energy and persistence conquer all things. ~Benjamin Franklin

My #1 FOCUS for today is:

Date:

Breakfast	Calories	Protein	Carbs	Fat	Sugar
Time:					
Totals					

Lunch	Calories	Protein	Carbs	Fat	Sugar
Time:					
Totals					

Dinner	Calories	Protein	Carbs	Fat	Sugar
Time:					
Totals					

Snacks	Calories	Protein	Carbs	Fat	Sugar
Time:					
Time:					
Time:					
Totals					

Daily Totals					

Water (4 ounces per square)																						
Protein (5 grams per square)																						
Vitamins (1 vitamin per square)																						
Exercise (10 minutes per square)																						

Was my #1 FOCUS accomplished today? Y ☐ N ☐ **My thoughts about today:**

Decide and fill-in your #1 FOCUS on tomorrow's page.

I am Decisive, Determined, Disciplined and Dynamic!

Day 66

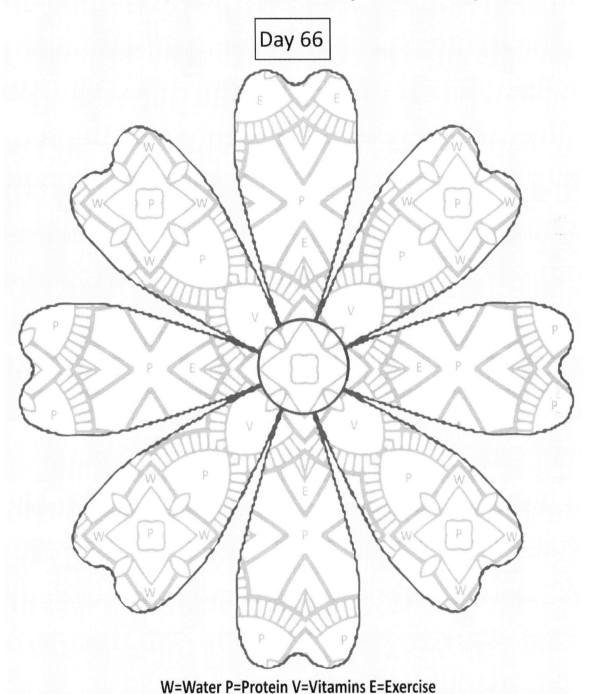

W=Water P=Protein V=Vitamins E=Exercise

THE BREAKTHROUGH JOURNAL

Nobody made a greater mistake than he who did nothing because he could do only a little. ~Edmund Burke

My #1 FOCUS for today is:

Date:

Breakfast	Calories	Protein	Carbs	Fat	Sugar
Time:					
Totals					

Lunch	Calories	Protein	Carbs	Fat	Sugar
Time:					
Totals					

Dinner	Calories	Protein	Carbs	Fat	Sugar
Time:					
Totals					

Snacks	Calories	Protein	Carbs	Fat	Sugar
Time:					
Time:					
Time:					
Totals					

Daily Totals					

Water (4 ounces per square)																					
Protein (5 grams per square)																					
Vitamins (1 vitamin per square)																					
Exercise (10 minutes per square)																					

Was my #1 FOCUS accomplished today? Y ☐ N ☐   My thoughts about today:

Decide and fill-in your #1 FOCUS on tomorrow's page.

I am Decisive, Determined, Disciplined and Dynamic!

Day 67

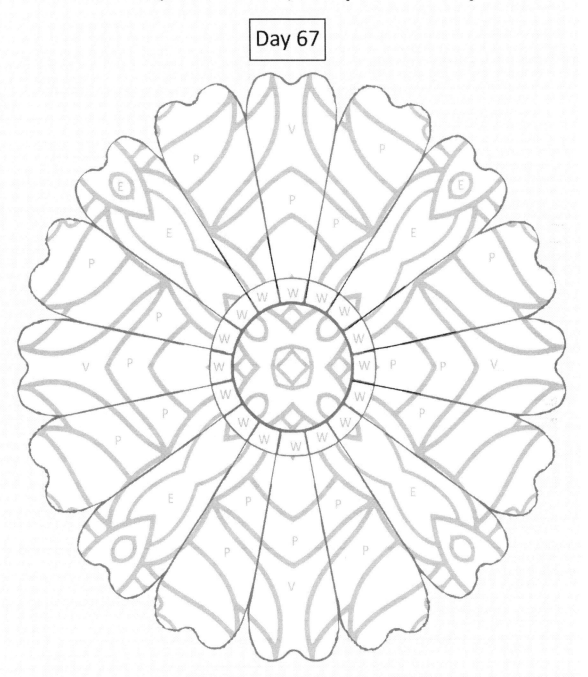

W=Water P=Protein V=Vitamins E=Exercise

THE BREAKTHROUGH JOURNAL

To reach a port, we must sail—Sail, not tie at anchor—Sail, not drift. ~Franklin Roosevelt

My #1 FOCUS for today is:

Date:

Breakfast	Calories	Protein	Carbs	Fat	Sugar
Time:					
Totals					

Lunch	Calories	Protein	Carbs	Fat	Sugar
Time:					
Totals					

Dinner	Calories	Protein	Carbs	Fat	Sugar
Time:					
Totals					

Snacks	Calories	Protein	Carbs	Fat	Sugar
Time:					
Time:					
Time:					
Totals					

Daily Totals					

Water (4 ounces per square)																
Protein (5 grams per square)																
Vitamins (1 vitamin per square)																
Exercise (10 minutes per square)																

Was my #1 FOCUS accomplished today? Y ☐ N ☐ My thoughts about today:

Decide and fill-in your #1 FOCUS on tomorrow's page.

THE BREAKTHROUGH JOURNAL

I am Decisive, Determined, Disciplined and Dynamic!

Day 68

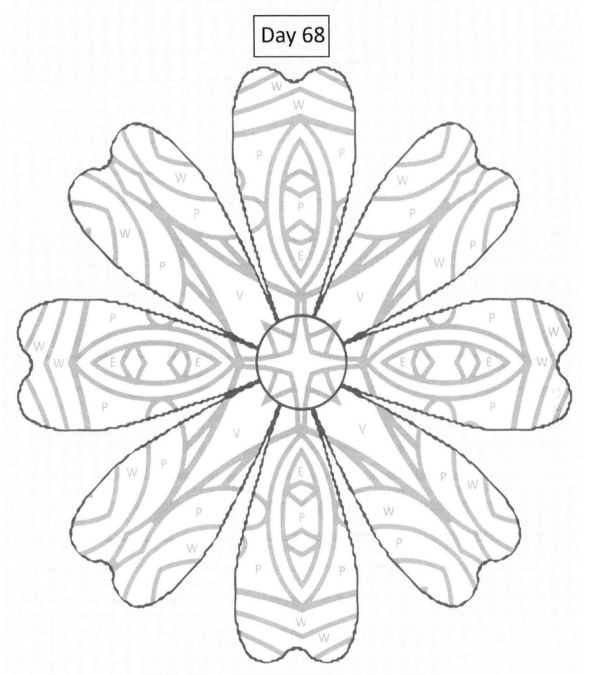

W=Water P=Protein V=Vitamins E=Exercise

THE BREAKTHROUGH JOURNAL

What lies behind us and what lies before us are tiny matters compared to what lies within us. ~Ralph Waldo Emerson

My #1 FOCUS for today is:

Date:

Breakfast	Calories	Protein	Carbs	Fat	Sugar
Time:					
Totals					

Lunch	Calories	Protein	Carbs	Fat	Sugar
Time:					
Totals					

Dinner	Calories	Protein	Carbs	Fat	Sugar
Time:					
Totals					

Snacks	Calories	Protein	Carbs	Fat	Sugar
Time:					
Time:					
Time:					
Totals					

Daily Totals					

Water (4 ounces per square)											
Protein (5 grams per square)											
Vitamins (1 vitamin per square)											
Exercise (10 minutes per square)											

Was my #1 FOCUS accomplished today? Y ☐ N ☐ My thoughts about today:

Decide and fill-in your #1 FOCUS on tomorrow's page.

THE BREAKTHROUGH JOURNAL

I am Decisive, Determined, Disciplined and Dynamic!

Day 69

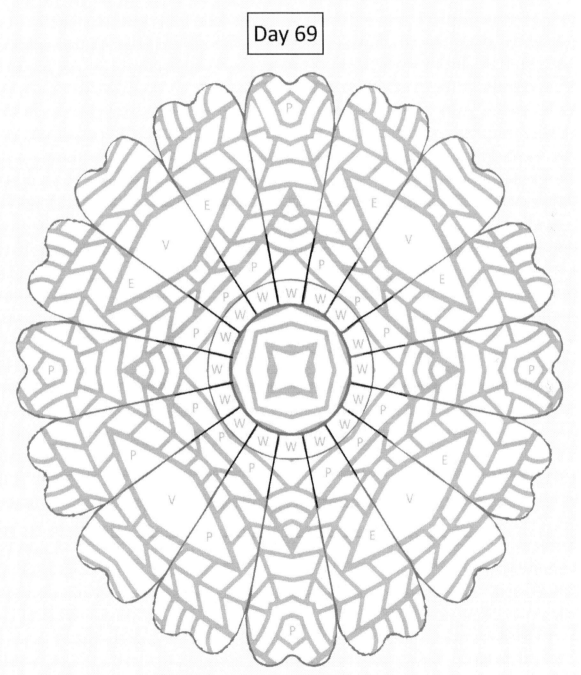

W=Water P=Protein V=Vitamins E=Exercise

THE BREAKTHROUGH JOURNAL

To gain self-respect, you need to put yourself first. ~Lorii Myers

My #1 FOCUS for today is:

Date:

Breakfast	Calories	Protein	Carbs	Fat	Sugar
Time:					
Totals					

Lunch	Calories	Protein	Carbs	Fat	Sugar
Time:					
Totals					

Dinner	Calories	Protein	Carbs	Fat	Sugar
Time:					
Totals					

Snacks	Calories	Protein	Carbs	Fat	Sugar
Time:					
Time:					
Time:					
Totals					

Daily Totals					

Water (4 ounces per square)														
Protein (5 grams per square)														
Vitamins (1 vitamin per square)														
Exercise (10 minutes per square)														

Was my #1 FOCUS accomplished today? Y ☐ N ☐ **My thoughts about today:**

Decide and fill-in your #1 FOCUS on tomorrow's page.

THE BREAKTHROUGH JOURNAL

I am Decisive, Determined, Disciplined and Dynamic!

Day 70

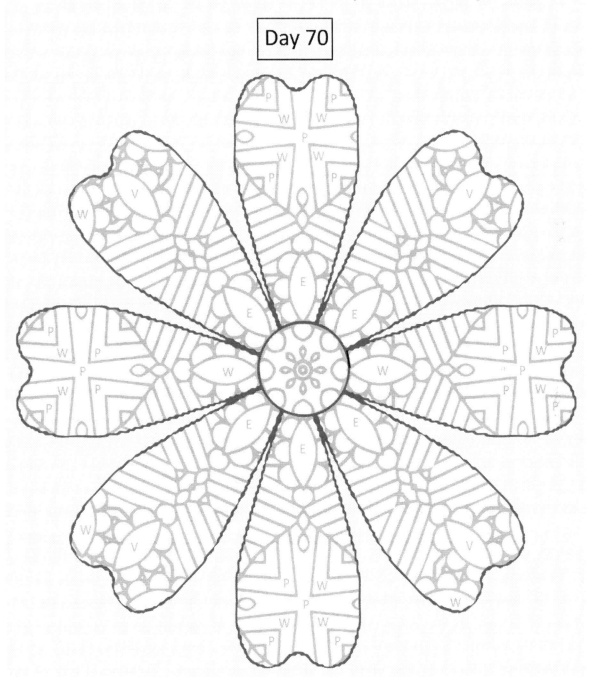

W=Water P=Protein V=Vitamins E=Exercise

WEEKLY REVIEW

Did I accomplish my goal this week?_____

What went well this week?_____

_____

_____

_____

What can be improved?_____

_____

_____

_____

My goal for the coming week is_____

_____

_____

My daily plan to accomplish this goal is_____

_____

_____

_____

_____

_____

This is the behavior I will change this week_____

_____

THOUGHTS & IDEAS

THE BREAKTHROUGH JOURNAL

Don't wait. The time will never be just right. ~Napoleon Hill

My #1 FOCUS for today is:

Date:

Breakfast	Calories	Protein	Carbs	Fat	Sugar
Time:					
Totals					

Lunch	Calories	Protein	Carbs	Fat	Sugar
Time:					
Totals					

Dinner	Calories	Protein	Carbs	Fat	Sugar
Time:					
Totals					

Snacks	Calories	Protein	Carbs	Fat	Sugar
Time:					
Time:					
Time:					
Totals					

Daily Totals					

Water (4 ounces per square)															
Protein (5 grams per square)															
Vitamins (1 vitamin per square)															
Exercise (10 minutes per square)															

Was my #1 FOCUS accomplished today? Y ☐ N ☐ **My thoughts about today:**

Decide and fill-in your #1 FOCUS on tomorrow's page.

I am Decisive, Determined, Disciplined and Dynamic!

Day 71

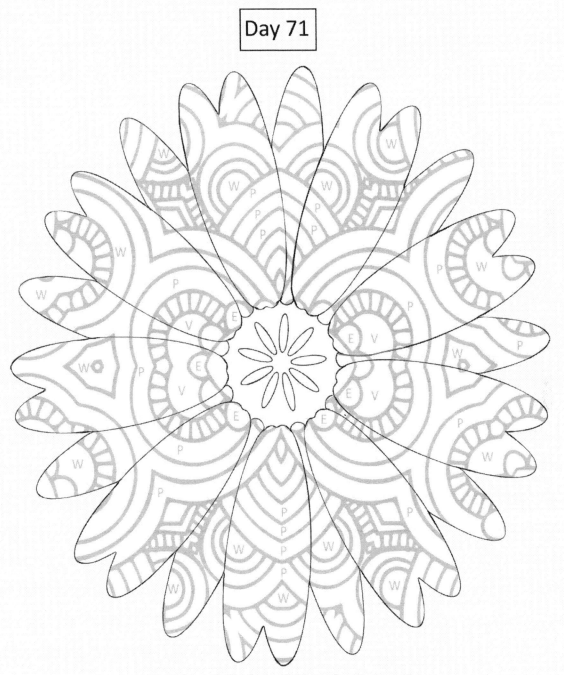

W=Water P=Protein V=Vitamins E=Exercise

THE BREAKTHROUGH JOURNAL

Attitude is a little thing that makes a big difference. ~Winston Churchill

My #1 FOCUS for today is:

Date:

Breakfast	Calories	Protein	Carbs	Fat	Sugar
Time:					
Totals					

Lunch	Calories	Protein	Carbs	Fat	Sugar
Time:					
Totals					

Dinner	Calories	Protein	Carbs	Fat	Sugar
Time:					
Totals					

Snacks	Calories	Protein	Carbs	Fat	Sugar
Time:					
Time:					
Time:					
Totals					

Daily Totals					

Water (4 ounces per square)																	
Protein (5 grams per square)																	
Vitamins (1 vitamin per square)																	
Exercise (10 minutes per square)																	

Was my #1 FOCUS accomplished today? Y ☐ N ☐ My thoughts about today:

Decide and fill-in your #1 FOCUS on tomorrow's page.

I am Decisive, Determined, Disciplined and Dynamic!

Day 72

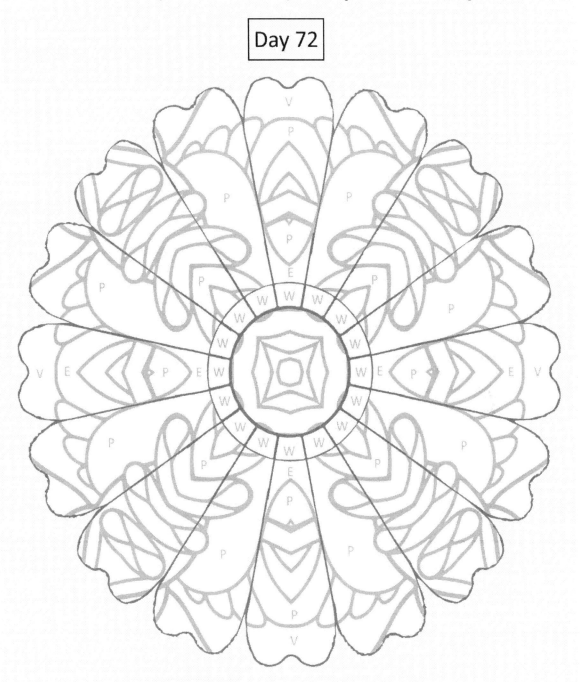

W=Water P=Protein V=Vitamins E=Exercise

THE BREAKTHROUGH JOURNAL

Show up in every single moment like you're meant to be there. ~Marie Forleo

My #1 FOCUS for today is:

Date:

Breakfast	Calories	Protein	Carbs	Fat	Sugar
Time:					
Totals					

Lunch	Calories	Protein	Carbs	Fat	Sugar
Time:					
Totals					

Dinner	Calories	Protein	Carbs	Fat	Sugar
Time:					
Totals					

Snacks	Calories	Protein	Carbs	Fat	Sugar
Time:					
Time:					
Time:					
Totals					

Daily Totals					

Water (4 ounces per square)																
Protein (5 grams per square)																
Vitamins (1 vitamin per square)																
Exercise (10 minutes per square)																

Was my #1 FOCUS accomplished today? Y ☐ N ☐ My thoughts about today:

Decide and fill-in your #1 FOCUS on tomorrow's page.

THE BREAKTHROUGH JOURNAL

I am Decisive, Determined, Disciplined and Dynamic!

Day 73

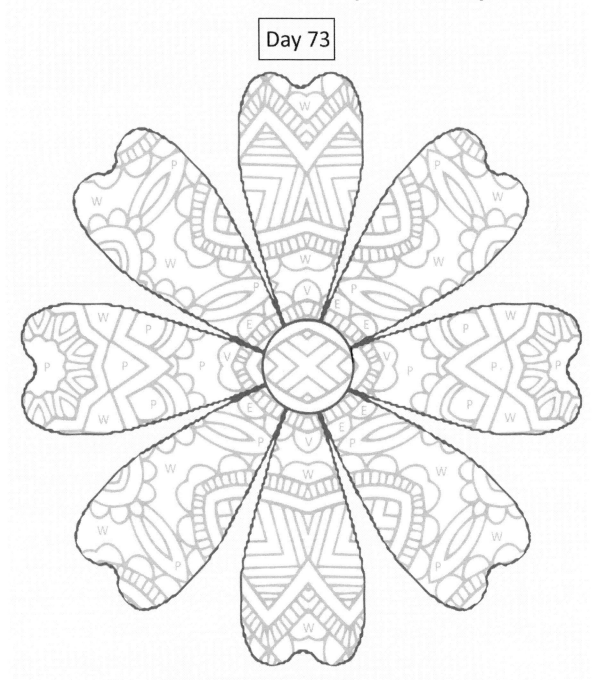

W=Water P=Protein V=Vitamins E=Exercise

THE BREAKTHROUGH JOURNAL

The grateful mind continually expects good things, and expectation becomes faith. ~Wallace D. Wattles

My #1 FOCUS for today is:

Date:

Breakfast	Calories	Protein	Carbs	Fat	Sugar
Time:					
Totals					

Lunch	Calories	Protein	Carbs	Fat	Sugar
Time:					
Totals					

Dinner	Calories	Protein	Carbs	Fat	Sugar
Time:					
Totals					

Snacks	Calories	Protein	Carbs	Fat	Sugar
Time:					
Time:					
Time:					
Totals					

Daily Totals					

Water (4 ounces per square)																	
Protein (5 grams per square)																	
Vitamins (1 vitamin per square)																	
Exercise (10 minutes per square)																	

Was my #1 FOCUS accomplished today? Y ☐ N ☐ My thoughts about today:

Decide and fill-in your #1 FOCUS on tomorrow's page.

THE BREAKTHROUGH JOURNAL

I am Decisive, Determined, Disciplined and Dynamic!

Day 74

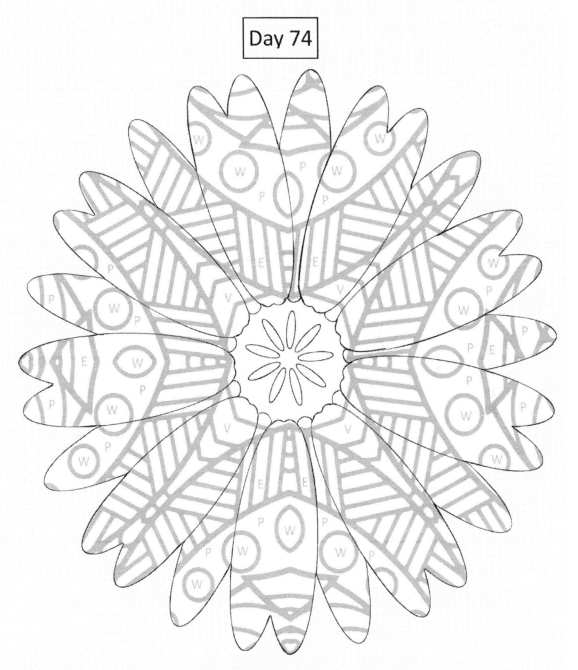

W=Water P=Protein V=Vitamins E=Exercise

THE BREAKTHROUGH JOURNAL

Don't let what you cannot do interfere with what you can do. ~John R. Wooden

My #1 FOCUS for today is:

Date:

Breakfast	Calories	Protein	Carbs	Fat	Sugar
Time:					
Totals					

Lunch	Calories	Protein	Carbs	Fat	Sugar
Time:					
Totals					

Dinner	Calories	Protein	Carbs	Fat	Sugar
Time:					
Totals					

Snacks	Calories	Protein	Carbs	Fat	Sugar
Time:					
Time:					
Time:					
Totals					

Daily Totals					

Water (4 ounces per square)																
Protein (5 grams per square)																
Vitamins (1 vitamin per square)																
Exercise (10 minutes per square)																

Was my #1 FOCUS accomplished today? Y ☐ N ☐ My thoughts about today:

Decide and fill-in your #1 FOCUS on tomorrow's page.

I am Decisive, Determined, Disciplined and Dynamic!

Day 75

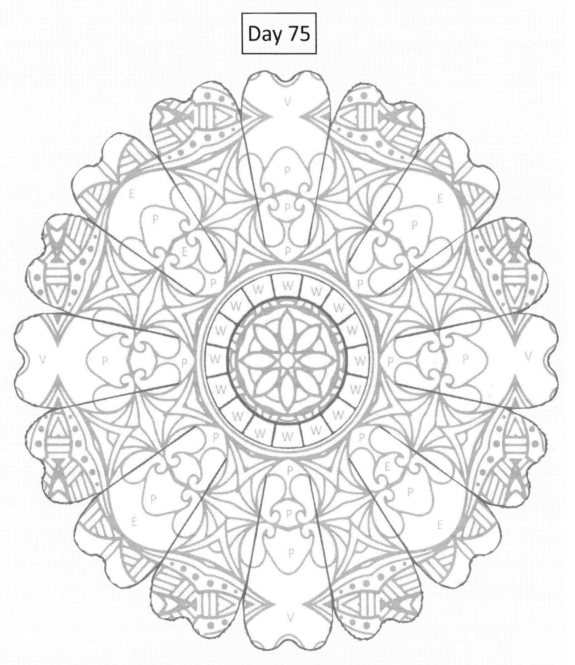

W=Water P=Protein V=Vitamins E=Exercise

THE BREAKTHROUGH JOURNAL

Believe that life is worth living and your belief will help create the fact. ~William James

My #1 FOCUS for today is:

Date:

Breakfast	Calories	Protein	Carbs	Fat	Sugar
Time:					
Totals					

Lunch	Calories	Protein	Carbs	Fat	Sugar
Time:					
Totals					

Dinner	Calories	Protein	Carbs	Fat	Sugar
Time:					
Totals					

Snacks	Calories	Protein	Carbs	Fat	Sugar
Time:					
Time:					
Time:					
Totals					

Daily Totals					

Water (4 ounces per square)																					
Protein (5 grams per square)																					
Vitamins (1 vitamin per square)																					
Exercise (10 minutes per square)																					

Was my #1 FOCUS accomplished today? Y ☐ N ☐ My thoughts about today:

Decide and fill-in your #1 FOCUS on tomorrow's page.

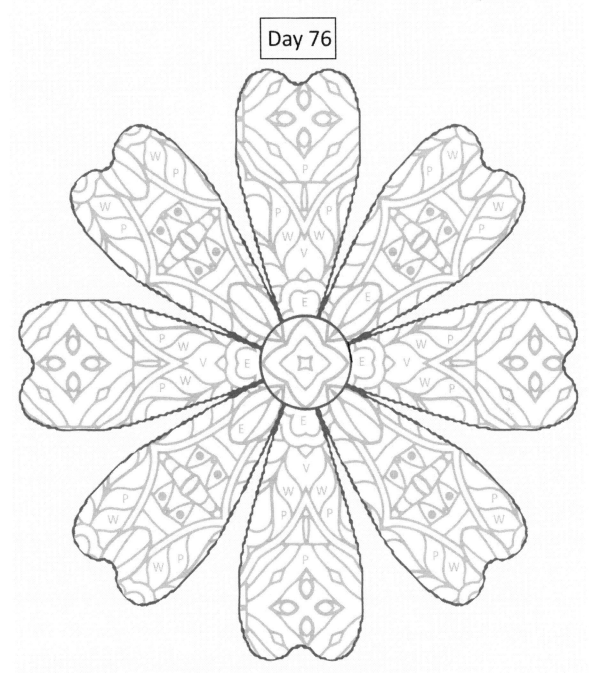

THE BREAKTHROUGH JOURNAL

I am Decisive, Determined, Disciplined and Dynamic!

Day 76

W=Water P=Protein V=Vitamins E=Exercise

THE BREAKTHROUGH JOURNAL

That some achieve great success, is proof to all that others can achieve it as well. ~Abraham Lincoln

My #1 FOCUS for today is:

Date:

Breakfast	Calories	Protein	Carbs	Fat	Sugar
Time:					
Totals					

Lunch	Calories	Protein	Carbs	Fat	Sugar
Time:					
Totals					

Dinner	Calories	Protein	Carbs	Fat	Sugar
Time:					
Totals					

Snacks	Calories	Protein	Carbs	Fat	Sugar
Time:					
Time:					
Time:					
Totals					

Daily Totals					

Water (4 ounces per square)																	
Protein (5 grams per square)																	
Vitamins (1 vitamin per square)																	
Exercise (10 minutes per square)																	

Was my #1 FOCUS accomplished today? Y ☐ N ☐ My thoughts about today:

Decide and fill-in your #1 FOCUS on tomorrow's page.

I am Decisive, Determined, Disciplined and Dynamic!

Day 77

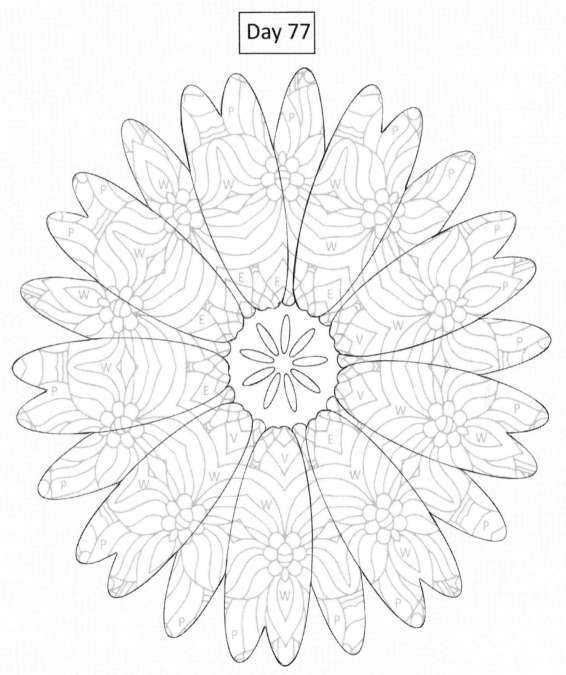

W=Water P=Protein V=Vitamins E=Exercise

WEEKLY REVIEW

Did I accomplish my goal this week?_____

What went well this week?_____
_____
_____
_____

What can be improved?_____
_____
_____
_____

My goal for the coming week is_____
_____
_____

My daily plan to accomplish this goal is_____
_____
_____
_____
_____
_____

This is the behavior I will change this week_____
_____

THOUGHTS & IDEAS

THE BREAKTHROUGH JOURNAL

Goals allow you to control the direction of change in your favor. ~Brian Tracy

My #1 FOCUS for today is:

Date:

Breakfast	Calories	Protein	Carbs	Fat	Sugar
Time:					
Totals					

Lunch	Calories	Protein	Carbs	Fat	Sugar
Time:					
Totals					

Dinner	Calories	Protein	Carbs	Fat	Sugar
Time:					
Totals					

Snacks	Calories	Protein	Carbs	Fat	Sugar
Time:					
Time:					
Time:					
Totals					

Daily Totals					

Water (4 ounces per square)																	
Protein (5 grams per square)																	
Vitamins (1 vitamin per square)																	
Exercise (10 minutes per square)																	

Was my #1 FOCUS accomplished today? Y ☐ N ☐ My thoughts about today:

Decide and fill-in your #1 FOCUS on tomorrow's page.

THE BREAKTHROUGH JOURNAL

I am Decisive, Determined, Disciplined and Dynamic!

Day 78

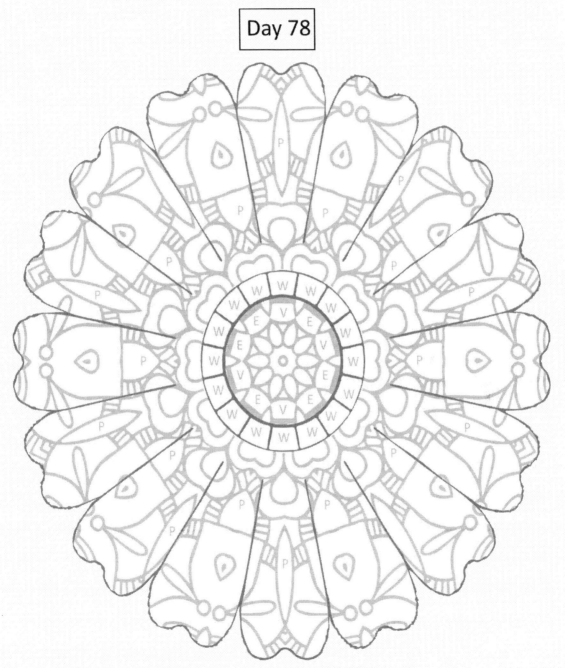

W=Water P=Protein V=Vitamins E=Exercise

THE BREAKTHROUGH JOURNAL

To quit is to fail - as long as you are still in the game you are succeeding! ~Lindsey Rietzsch

My #1 FOCUS for today is:
Date:

Breakfast	Calories	Protein	Carbs	Fat	Sugar
Time:					
Totals					

Lunch	Calories	Protein	Carbs	Fat	Sugar
Time:					
Totals					

Dinner	Calories	Protein	Carbs	Fat	Sugar
Time:					
Totals					

Snacks	Calories	Protein	Carbs	Fat	Sugar
Time:					
Time:					
Time:					
Totals					

Daily Totals					

Water (4 ounces per square)																
Protein (5 grams per square)																
Vitamins (1 vitamin per square)																
Exercise (10 minutes per square)																

Was my #1 FOCUS accomplished today? Y ☐ N ☐ **My thoughts about today:**

Decide and fill-in your #1 FOCUS on tomorrow's page.

THE BREAKTHROUGH JOURNAL

I am Decisive, Determined, Disciplined and Dynamic!

Day 79

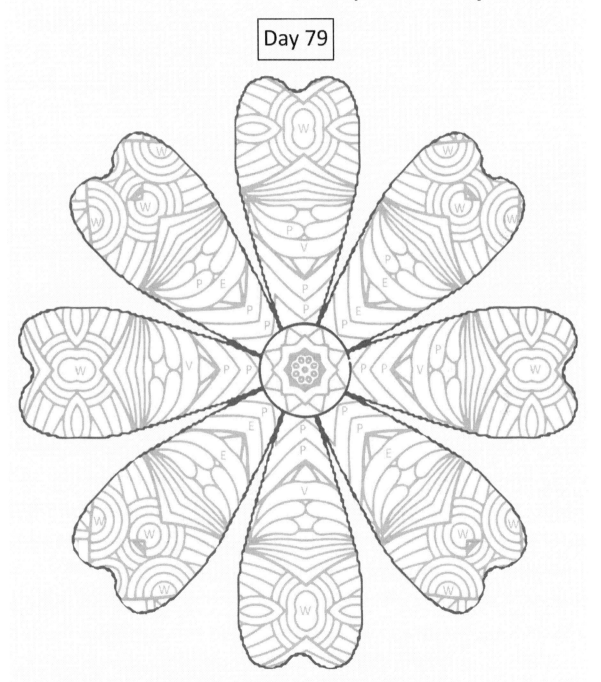

W=Water P=Protein V=Vitamins E=Exercise

THE BREAKTHROUGH JOURNAL

Just breathe and believe. ~Jodi Livon

My #1 FOCUS for today is:

Date:

Breakfast	Calories	Protein	Carbs	Fat	Sugar
Time:					
Totals					

Lunch	Calories	Protein	Carbs	Fat	Sugar
Time:					
Totals					

Dinner	Calories	Protein	Carbs	Fat	Sugar
Time:					
Totals					

Snacks	Calories	Protein	Carbs	Fat	Sugar
Time:					
Time:					
Time:					
Totals					

Daily Totals					

Water (4 ounces per square)																
Protein (5 grams per square)																
Vitamins (1 vitamin per square)																
Exercise (10 minutes per square)																

Was my #1 FOCUS accomplished today? Y ☐ N ☐ **My thoughts about today:**

Decide and fill-in your #1 FOCUS on tomorrow's page.

I am Decisive, Determined, Disciplined and Dynamic!

Day 80

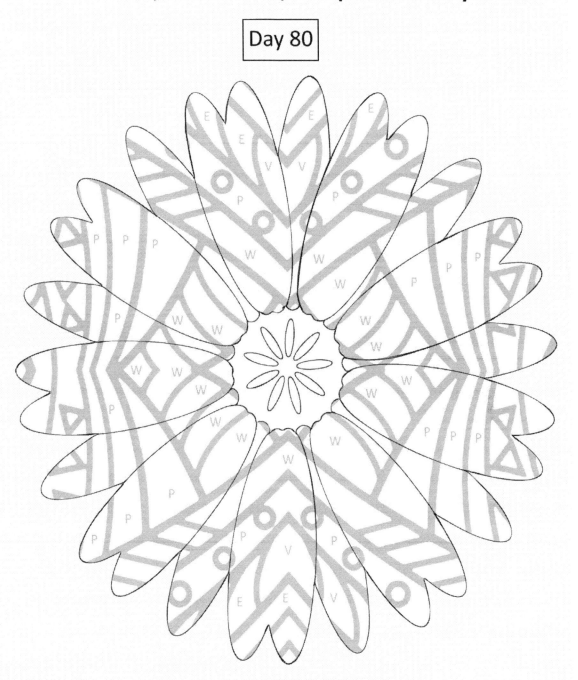

W=Water P=Protein V=Vitamins E=Exercise

THE BREAKTHROUGH JOURNAL

It is never too late to be what you might have been. ~George Eliot

My #1 FOCUS for today is:

Date:

Breakfast	Calories	Protein	Carbs	Fat	Sugar
Time:					
Totals					

Lunch	Calories	Protein	Carbs	Fat	Sugar
Time:					
Totals					

Dinner	Calories	Protein	Carbs	Fat	Sugar
Time:					
Totals					

Snacks	Calories	Protein	Carbs	Fat	Sugar
Time:					
Time:					
Time:					
Totals					

Daily Totals					

Water (4 ounces per square)																
Protein (5 grams per square)																
Vitamins (1 vitamin per square)																
Exercise (10 minutes per square)																

Was my #1 FOCUS accomplished today? Y ☐ N ☐ **My thoughts about today:**

Decide and fill-in your #1 FOCUS on tomorrow's page.

THE BREAKTHROUGH JOURNAL

I am Decisive, Determined, Disciplined and Dynamic!

Day 81

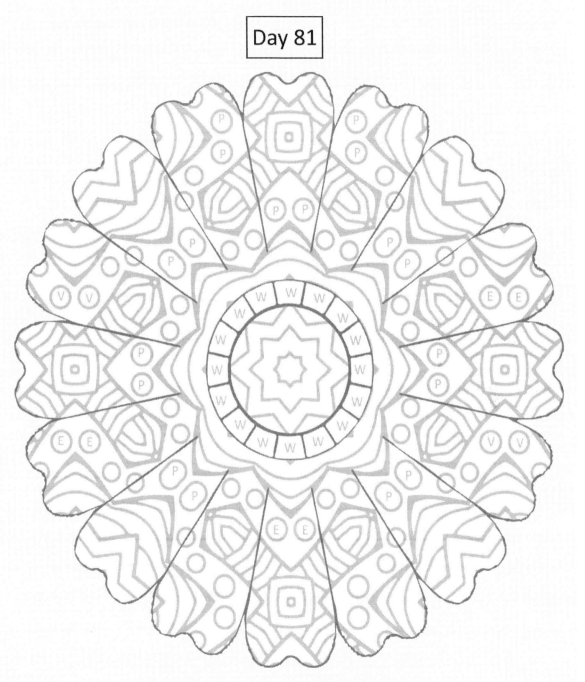

W=Water P=Protein V=Vitamins E=Exercise

THE BREAKTHROUGH JOURNAL

"You were designed, from birth, to succeed." ~Dr. Shad Helmstetter

My #1 FOCUS for today is:

Date:

Breakfast	Calories	Protein	Carbs	Fat	Sugar
Time:					
Totals					

Lunch	Calories	Protein	Carbs	Fat	Sugar
Time:					
Totals					

Dinner	Calories	Protein	Carbs	Fat	Sugar
Time:					
Totals					

Snacks	Calories	Protein	Carbs	Fat	Sugar
Time:					
Time:					
Time:					
Totals					

Daily Totals					

Water (4 ounces per square)																
Protein (5 grams per square)																
Vitamins (1 vitamin per square)																
Exercise (10 minutes per square)																

Was my #1 FOCUS accomplished today? Y ☐ N ☐ **My thoughts about today:**

Decide and fill-in your #1 FOCUS on tomorrow's page.

I am Decisive, Determined, Disciplined and Dynamic!

Day 82

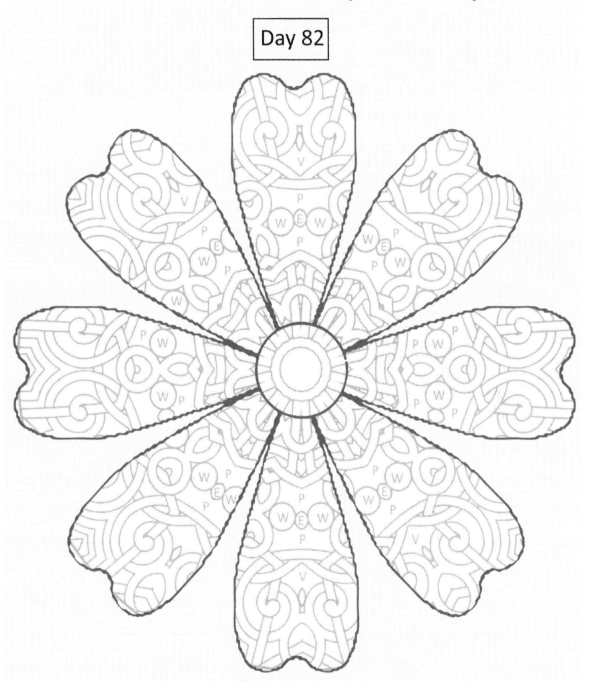

W=Water P=Protein V=Vitamins E=Exercise

THE BREAKTHROUGH JOURNAL

I have found that if you love life, life will love you back. ~Arthur Rubinstein

My #1 FOCUS for today is:

Date:

Breakfast	Calories	Protein	Carbs	Fat	Sugar
Time:					
Totals					

Lunch	Calories	Protein	Carbs	Fat	Sugar
Time:					
Totals					

Dinner	Calories	Protein	Carbs	Fat	Sugar
Time:					
Totals					

Snacks	Calories	Protein	Carbs	Fat	Sugar
Time:					
Time:					
Time:					
Totals					

Daily Totals					

Water (4 ounces per square)											
Protein (5 grams per square)											
Vitamins (1 vitamin per square)											
Exercise (10 minutes per square)											

Was my #1 FOCUS accomplished today? Y ☐ N ☐ My thoughts about today:

Decide and fill-in your #1 FOCUS on tomorrow's page.

214

THE BREAKTHROUGH JOURNAL

I am Decisive, Determined, Disciplined and Dynamic!

Day 83

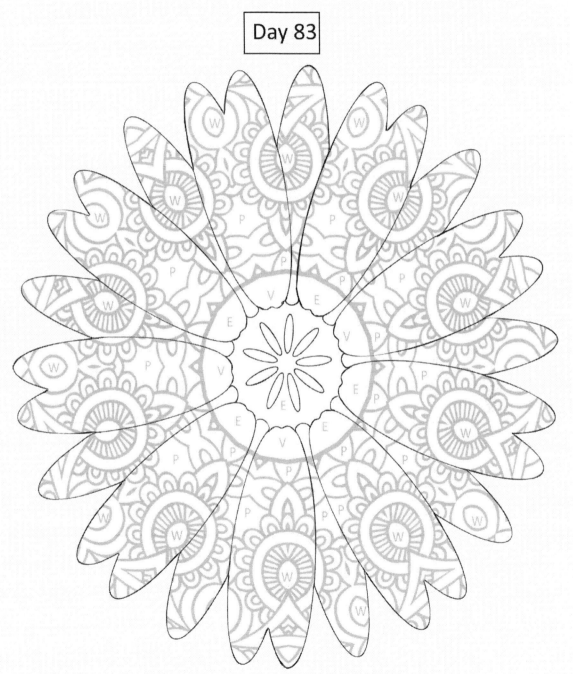

W=Water P=Protein V=Vitamins E=Exercise

THE BREAKTHROUGH JOURNAL

Life is a journey of learning and adapting. ~Beth Bianca

My #1 FOCUS for today is:

Date:

Breakfast	Calories	Protein	Carbs	Fat	Sugar
Time:					
Totals					

Lunch	Calories	Protein	Carbs	Fat	Sugar
Time:					
Totals					

Dinner	Calories	Protein	Carbs	Fat	Sugar
Time:					
Totals					

Snacks	Calories	Protein	Carbs	Fat	Sugar
Time:					
Time:					
Time:					
Totals					

Daily Totals					

Water (4 ounces per square)																				
Protein (5 grams per square)																				
Vitamins (1 vitamin per square)																				
Exercise (10 minutes per square)																				

Was my #1 FOCUS accomplished today? Y ☐ N ☐ My thoughts about today:

Decide and fill-in your #1 FOCUS on tomorrow's page.

I am Decisive, Determined, Disciplined and Dynamic!

Day 84

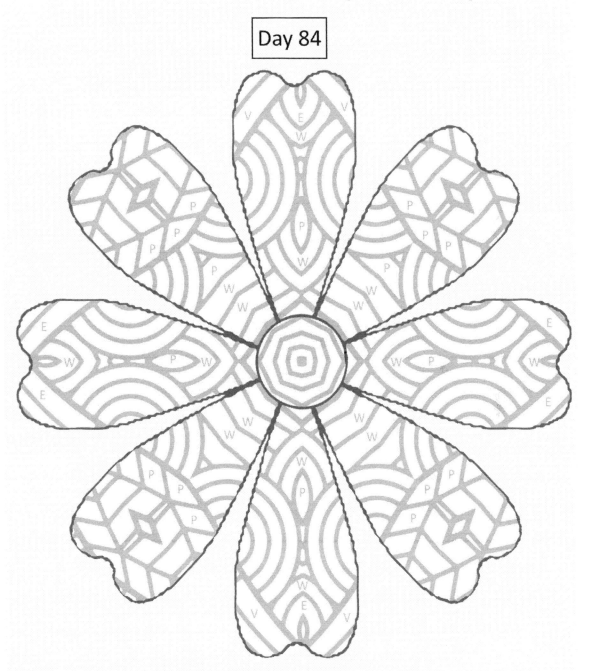

W=Water P=Protein V=Vitamins E=Exercise

WEEKLY REVIEW

Did I accomplish my goal this week?_____

_____

What went well this week?_____

_____

_____

_____

_____

_____

What can be improved?_____

_____

_____

_____

_____

AFTER STATS

Date:_____

Weight:_____

Bust Measurement:_____

Hips Measurement:_____

Record your After Stats on page 24.
Take an After Photo and tape it to page 25.

THE BREAKTHROUGH JOURNAL

12-WEEK REVIEW

Did I stick to my plan and accomplish my Breakthrough Goal?_____

_____

My major accomplishments during the last 12 weeks are_____

_____

_____

_____

_____

This is how my life has changed during the last 12 weeks_____

_____

_____

_____

_____

_____

_____

This is what I've learned about myself during the last 12 weeks_____

_____

_____

_____

_____

_____

THOUGHTS & IDEAS

THOUGHTS & IDEAS

BIBLIOGRAPHY

[Ref- 1]

http://www.webmd.com/diet/news/20080708/keeping-food-diary-helps-lose-weight

[Ref- 2]

http://www.fooducate.com/app#!page=post&id=57A352A4-5D18-87FE-404D-B75546CD8EB3

[Ref- 3]

http://www.medicaldaily.com/therapeutic-science-adult-coloring-books-how-childhood-pastime-helps-adults-356280

[Ref- 4]

http://www.huffingtonpost.com/dr-nikki-martinez-psyd-lcpc/7-reasons-adult-coloring-books-are-great-for-your-mental-emotional-and-intellectual-health_b_8626136.html

[Ref- 5]

http://www.riversideonline.com/employees/myhealthylifestyle/newsletter/half-hour-window.cfm?RenderForPrint=1

[Ref– 6]

http://bariatrics.ucla.edu/workfiles/UCLA-Bariatric-postoperative-diet-instructions.pdf

[Ref- 7]

http://www.hopkinsmedicine.org/johns_hopkins_bayview/_docs/medical_services/bariatrics/nutrition_weight_loss_surgery.pdf

[Ref- 8]

http://www.bariatric-surgery-source.com/bariatric-diet.html#4._Drink

[Ref- 9]

http://www.heart.org/HEARTORG/HealthyLiving/PhysicalActivity/FitnessBasics/American

-Heart-Association-Recommendations-for-Physical-Activity-in-

Adults_UCM_307976_Article.jsp#.V_RDJPkrJdi

[Ref-10]

http://www.obesitycoverage.com/gastric-sleeve-referencemanual/

[Ref- 11]

http://www.everydayhealth.com/weight/busting-the-muscle-weighs-more-than-fat-

myth.aspx

 [Ref- 12]

https://asmbs.org/patients/life-after-bariatric-surgery

ABOUT THE AUTHOR

Beth Bianca is a bariatric patient who lost 229 pounds. She is the author of *Mindset Breakthrough: Achieve Weight-Loss Surgery Success* and *The Breakthrough Journal: Butterfly Edition*. Beth is the founder of LadiesInWeighting.com, and a contributing author to the Huffington Post.

After weighing 394 pounds and becoming riddled with health issues, Beth received a second chance at life by having weight-loss surgery. She is passionate about sharing the lessons she has learned and providing support to other bariatric patients.

Beth is a Certified Life Coach and Lifestyle & Weight Management Specialist. You can find her at **BethBianca.com** and connect with her on **Facebook.com/BethBianca.Author/**

Receive notifications of new releases and special offers by simply using your phone.

Text the word **LIVING** to **444999**.

Other Books by Beth Bianca

Mindset Breakthrough: *Achieve Weight-Loss Surgery Success*

The Breakthrough Journal: *Butterfly Edition*

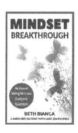 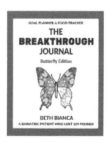

Visit the Butterfly Warrior Shop

T-Shirts, Hoodies, Mugs, and More

BethBianca.com/Shop/

Made in the USA
Lexington, KY
30 September 2017